Prai

'Sarah-Anne Lucas (Bird) is honest, direct and committed to helping you optimise your health and have more energy, a better relationship with your health and a better life. She wants you to eat better, be more flexible and have greater mobility and range. But be warned, *It's Never About The Fitness* requires you to participate. As you will discover, why you want to be healthier, fitter, in shape and more energised (the mindset) is foundational and more important that the workouts and the diet. Sarah has nursing qualification think or feel they have had enough. If her approach works for them it will definitely work for you. From the very get-go, *It's Never About The Fitness* is powerful, thought provoking and engaging; a habit-shifting starting point.

Andrew Priestley MD, The Coaching Experience (UK)

'Sarah's words are filled with love, compassion and encouragement, and reading them it would be impossible for anyone not to want more – and better – for themselves, no matter what state their life is currently in. Her story is one that many others have experienced in varying degrees and shades, and this makes it easy to grasp the idea that her triumph is something that anyone can have. This book will embrace you with Sarah's kindness, strength and energy until you can generate your own, in overflowing amounts, for yourself and for others.'

Michael Serwa, Author and Life Coach

'*It's Never About The Fitness* opens you to a mindset that is empowering, informative and based on real experience. As you read through the pages, you can't but help falling in love with the author's desire to help others. A powerful book which I would recommend you read. When I read it it felt as if I was talking to Sarah. The section about feeling needed was raw, honest, touching.'

Darshana Ubl, Small Business Advisor, Entrepreneur

'I've Known Sarah for over two years now and even when she claims to be having a less-than-good day she is vibrant and full of an infectious energy. She lives by the principles shared in her book. She treats her body with a respect that I truly envy. From her, I have learnt that energy is holistic, it's not just about rituals but the nourishment we provide our bodies. Take her words to heart and you will transform not just your body but your life.

Heather Katsonga Woodward, Founder of NenoNatural.com, the biggest UK blog for kinky and curly hair

'"Habits Maketh Man." How great to have such effective and easy to follow habits listed. Easy to follow instructions for a better life.'

Jane Alton, the UK's No. 1 Numerologist

'There are some people in the world who influence and persuade others temporarily. Then there is Sarah-Anne Lucas who has influence and persuasion so huge and effective it changes people's lives permanently! In this book Sarah shares simple yet profound ideas; she calls them rituals for every day. These rituals are simple but massively effective. She will show you what she has done for herself, what actually works and will help you find your amazing self. This book embodies Sarah's passion and genuine energy for life. Reading this book will help you to change yourself dramatically for the better. The way that Sarah writes and delivers her incredible knowledge and wisdom will help you to implement positive changes day by day until, by the end of the book, you may not recognise your old self. So if you are ready to transition and become the amazing person you only dream of being, read this book! Sarah has a positively infectious personality which leaps out of the pages saying to you, "Come with me, let me show you how you can be extraordinary, beautiful and incredible!" Once you get started you won't want to stop and your life will never be the same again.'

Aly Harrold, Coaching for Public Speaking, www.alyharrold.co.uk

'In *It's Never About The Fitness* you are introduced to cutting edge information and techniques that anyone can use to get moving and motivated to move well. These skills will give you tools to encourage proactive self-care, support and encouragement.

'I love Sarah's simple and practical approach to supporting women in health. Sarah uses real people's breaking point, their 'Had Enough' moment, to show you we are all human. We all get those moments, it's how we move forward that paves the way to our health and happiness.

'The importance of her work relies on careful attention to the needs of the body and mind, and having built a safe, practical, universally accessible application. Sarah's programme, as laid out for you in *It's Never About The Fitness,* brings this to you in an easy, readable form. Enjoy your journey.'

Paul Massey B.A (Hons), M.C.S.P., S.R.P., Author of *Sports Pilates... How to Prevent and Overcome Sports Injuries*

'Reading Bird's book is like being bathed in sunlight: warm, cheering, positive. I'm a corporate animal – professional, time-poor and cynical about all the health and wellbeing tosh. Yet Sarah's book showed me how to get the best out of my physical capabilities and mind-set. With her three-step process and easy-to-follow daily rituals, I'm developing good habits that are making me healthier, stronger and fitter. Who knew that drinking 200 ml of water and taking pre-breakfast exercise for 20 minutes every day could make such a difference?! If I can do these, so can anyone. If you're an over-worked business-woman or a stressed-out, always on-the-go mum, (or more likely both), this book is for you!'

Henry Rose Lee, Author, Speaker, CEO of Talenttio,
International Business Mentor

Contents

'The beauty of a woman must be seen from in her eyes, because that is the doorway to her heart, the place where love resides.'

Audrey Hepburn

'Where there is a woman
there is magic.'

Ntozake Shange

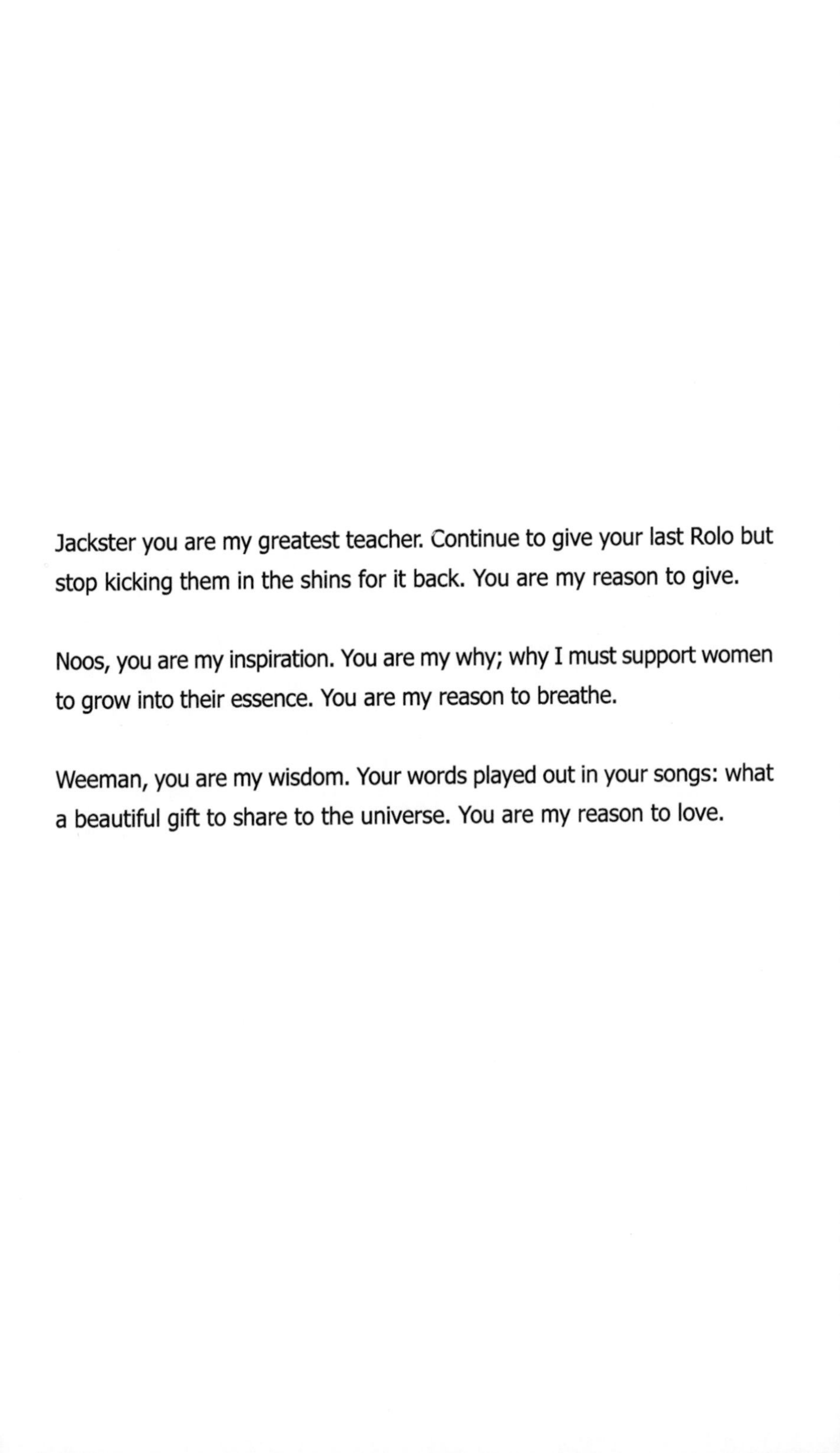

Jackster you are my greatest teacher. Continue to give your last Rolo but stop kicking them in the shins for it back. You are my reason to give.

Noos, you are my inspiration. You are my why; why I must support women to grow into their essence. You are my reason to breathe.

Weeman, you are my wisdom. Your words played out in your songs: what a beautiful gift to share to the universe. You are my reason to love.

Preface

'Stop eating, Fatty,' said in an American accent.

'That's mean, Bird!' I hear you say, but it's true.

Have I got your attention? Good. I say this with a cheeky smile and an intention of love, respect and excitement.

What if I could share with you the key to unlocking more energy than you could contain? So much energy that waking up couldn't come soon enough? You might still wake up tired – let's be real – but you would not want to hit the snooze button or dread the day ahead. What if I could give you daily rituals to create so much energy that it made you feel like you could burst? So much energy that you had to sing as loud as you could sat in your car, catching the eye of other drivers and making them laugh and smile, wishing that they were as effervescent as you. So much energy that you had to say hello to everyone who walked by you.

What if I could share with you the key to fat loss? You don't need to go to the gym.

'Woohoo!' I hear you say.

You don't need to wait to exercise until the squids have gone to school. You don't need to organise a babysitter to enjoy putting goodness into your body. You don't need to go to 'Fat Club' (not my description).

You never – yes, you heard right – need to jump on scales to weigh yourself. Let me repeat that: You will never need to weigh yourself.

What if I could share with you the key to diets (urgh, I hate that word 'diet') food intake, fuel, meals, goodness, nutrition... etc? You don't follow a points system. You don't follow a food-combining regime. You don't calorie count. You don't weigh your food. I could carry on, but as my nan used to say, 'If 'ifs' and 'ands' were pots and pans, there'd be no need for tinkers.'

Yes I can... do all of the above and so much more, All through simple one per cent tweaks to your daily activities.

This book is the beginning of your journey with Birdonabike. My name is Sarah-Anne, aka 'Bird'. All my friends and family call me 'Bird'; I would love you to do the same. I am from the West Country in England and we talk with a beautiful twang to our speech. When I moved to the South East of England, they picked up my 'Oh Arr' accent and nicknamed me 'Bird'. Twenty years on and it has stuck. Even my children call me 'Bird', when they can't get an answer to 'Mumma'. So I shared the love with the name of my company. It always makes me smile.

I will share with you all I know, and give you the belief to transition into being your best, every day.

This book will provide simple step-by-step advice and tips that can be easily incorporated into your Activities of Daily Living (ADLs).

Why is the book called 'It's Never About The Fitness'?

I support people to believe in their health. This has attracted women and men who had specific races they wanted to train for: Iron Man, marathons, triathlons, 10ks and Race for Life. Women in particular would ask for my support in devising a marathon plan, for example, or a 10k plan, and I would train them up for race day. From the first meeting it became apparent to me that running a race was never the result they were searching for. It was the sense of achievement and self-worth that would come from completing the task. They felt that running a race would give them what they yearned for: self-respect and respect from others, especially partners or husbands, a sense of pride in the achievement; and self-love. Once they had completed the race these feelings subsided and their previous emptiness returned, leaving them to continue the quest for self-fulfillment in the external environment rather than searching within. Racing broke their bodies, mentally and physically, instead of building them up. Exercise added another external stressor, which increased their toxic thoughts about themselves and deepened their fatigue.

It was at this point that I created my three-step approach to assessing personal energy.

Step 1 – Your thoughts
Step 2 – Your environment
Step 3 – Your nutrition

Only when all three steps have been addressed are we fit for fitness.

My approach takes real problems, faced by real women, in real time and in real people's environments, and looks at the biggest barriers to change in our lives.

What do humans want from their bodies, and how can I support them on their quest? This has become my daily waking obsession.

Introduction

'I'm where I'm meant to be.'

Rapunzel, *Tangled*

The Birdonabike story

Birdonabike evolved from losing everything (well, that's how I felt): my adored career, my second marriage and the life I had fooled myself into loving.

I had the most wonderful career in nursing, respected, valued and loved by my colleagues in a GP's surgery. We were implementing a new way of practising in the community. Nurses were growing in their role, diagnosing and prescribing, referring onwards, and dealing with minor injuries and illnesses, enabling the doctors to concentrate on chronic disease. I was flourishing as I prepared to start my master's degree, which was being piloted and assessed by the local authorities and the nurse training university.

At home, though, it was the complete opposite: my eldest son had been newly diagnosed with ADHD, autism and Tourette's; my second marriage was challenging – the love was there but the bricks in the wall were slowly falling out, and bringing children together from previous marriages with very unsupportive ex-partners was proving very difficult.

I hope I'm getting across to you the pain and anguish that I was going through. To be disliked, maybe even hated by the children of the blended family is hard to endure. But endurance is exactly the element of fitness

I encompassed. It was not the person the children hated, but the role I was forced to take. It was so sad to see the children's inner turmoil. 'Killing with kindness' may have been my wonderful mantra that I live by, but kindness was not what the children perceived.

I had no option but to support my family.

I resigned from the job I loved; I handed my husband my independence and finances, and every decision about my life. My focus became finding the correct schooling for Jack, and giving myself to my marriage. No way was I going to have a second failed marriage. One was enough for any lifetime.

Now my family was thriving, but where had I gone? This strong, financially independent, respected, adored, intelligent woman. *Gone*. I felt like I had sold my soul to the devil. I lost control; I was not even allowed to buy a CD that I loved. Listen to the language I'm using, 'allowed' and 'lost'. The truth is, I had relinquished my control; I had given it over, handed it on a plate to others. The only thing I could control was the food I put in my mouth. I became ill.

My poor family, my poor husband, my poor friends! Funnily enough, the children had no idea I had an eating disorder – well, I have always presumed they never knew.

I became a liar, not going to eating disorder clinic, taking laxatives, taking refuge in exercise, fooling everyone daily yet shrinking before their eyes. I had no idea that people could see this wonderful woman wasting away. Some friends flattered me with words of 'Wow, you're looking tiny' or 'Where have you gone?' – this was nectar to me. My aim was never to look skinny, thin or to lose weight; it was merely to disappear – and if I'm honest, to stick two fingers up to life, internally chanting, 'You can't control this part of my life'.

I can remember one day when it had all got too much. I left the house – with the children and my husband oblivious to me leaving – and drove away. No idea where I was going. Apparently, I drove for hours. Honestly, I can't remember much about this episode. I found myself sitting in a layby, unaware of the time, or of my reasons for leaving. Numb. I returned to the house. My husband asked no questions and I have never understood why not. Was he uncaring, or ignorant of what I had done, or did he feel that if he did not feed the behaviour it would go away. If I'm honest, he was damned if he did and damned if he didn't.

Ignorance and denial, I later found out, would be two of the greatest reasons for the failure of our marriage. Please hear this: Ignorance is Never Bliss.

But the tipping point came. I went to a meeting with my husband and sat in a room with young girls and their parents expressing their thoughts. I said nothing. All I had was a question to myself: 'What am I doing here?' My issues were never related to weight, or looks, just control. This moment sitting in a room, looking at these young girls and their family battles, was my 'had enough' moment.

Your 'had enough' moment will come too. You may think it already has. My guess is that you do think you have had enough, but your actions or behaviours are not yet aligned with your mindset.

How to use this book

This book is designed to offer simple tips and tweaks to your daily routines, but ones that will empower you to be your daily best. These tweaks may look simple to you, but they may not be that easy to implement on a consistent daily basis. Once you have made them part of your daily routine, though, your energy will be uncontainable. Your purpose will be defined and you will find the entry point to your continuous life journey.

'Teach thy tongue to say "I do not know", and thou shalt progress.'

Maimonides, Spanish philosopher (1135–1204)

You are now right where you should be: being courageous, being powerful in your learning process.

The four-step circle framework

I have created a simple four-step circle framework to be used within each chapter.

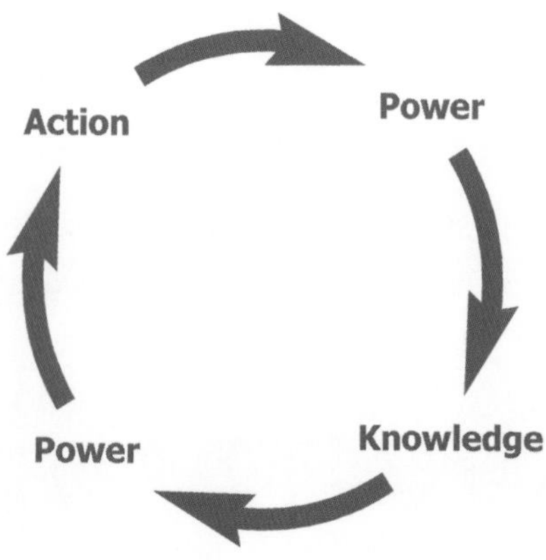

It is an ever-expanding circle. A continuum. Your starting point is wherever you find yourself in the circle, but my suggestion is you are in 'Power'. You must be. You have found the power within you to ask for more from yourself.

Once you have found the power to create forward movement in your life, you need the knowledge of how to do it. In each chapter there are actions to be completed. I will give you daily rituals to create structure and an abundance of energy. These rituals have a massive impact on your physiology and mindset. They are simple, but not necessarily easy. I have the greatest respect for you as you build the knowledge and power to action these rituals. My friends, you may try and fail many times. I'm telling you this so that when these episodes happen, you will be ready to move into 'Power' again, to re-energize feeling strong so that you can action the rituals again. You will proceed by little wins not quantum leaps. Be prepared to go back and forth along this spectrum; make this elastic band effect part of the journey. Take note: the quantum leap to success is there to be taken; it's not a question of 'will it happen?', it's just when.

You are high achievers. I know this, because you are reading this book. Everybody has great ideas but few act on those ideas. Many great ideas remain in words, circling the universe. They've been spoken but never actioned. You will take your power and knowledge to the next level. You will action your ideas. This is a must. Trust in this process. This is your time shine.

Make a note of each little win. Describe your feelings, your thoughts and actions. 'I've already been on immense journeys,' I hear you say. I do get it, I hear you. Hold on to these words. They are powerful. You have power within that you can tap in to, and I will guide you.

Equipment needed

- A notepad/journal chosen specifically to inspire you to record thoughts, feelings, achievements and results. (You're excited, just like back in those first days at school. Ah, the smell of a new book.)
- The right colour pen. (I will only write in blue. It shows my rebellious side: when I was a nurse, we were only allowed to use black, so every time I write in blue, it makes me chuckle.)
- A rebounder/mini trampoline
- A blender, juicer or Nutribullet
- A Japanese body brush
- An exercise mat
- An organic source for meat and vegetables – research local producers. (Livelean.co.uk are awesome. Tell them Birdonabike sent you.)

ACTION

This takes 2 minutes.

Here are three questions that will get you started on your first page:

1. Where am I now, at this very moment?
2. What do I want my life to look like? My future vision.
3. What resources do I need to get me there?

These are mindset changing questions. Super-powerful lifelong questions that can be applied to everything. These are inter-generational questions: you can teach your children to ask these questions throughout their lives, passing them on through the generations.

You will find this truly challenging: you may find you just sit there with nothing coming into your head, other than your negative internal chatter persuading you that this is a waste of your time.

You will return to these questions throughout this book.

'How does she know?' That's another question that you will repeat throughout this book, another question your negative internal chatter will challenge you with. I know because even now the negative internal chatter challenges me. I hear and acknowledge, pause, then power through and make the best decision.

The negative internal chatter encourages you to make decisions that may not be in your best interest.

Notice I did not say 'bad'. There are no bad decisions. The decisions you make are made with the information you have to hand at that time. Every decision you make is made with respect and love, and aims to achieve the best result, but hindsight is a wonderful thing.

Gabrielle Bernstein calls her internal chatter 'ing'. 'Ing' is your ego. I love that. We all have internal chatter going on all day. Some perceive it as voices, devils on shoulders, or their naughty side. The perception of internal dialogue is varied.

We all have an ego, but some have grown bigger than others. Some live with their ego, some are controlled by their ego and others love their ego. Having an ego is exciting. It keeps you disciplined, aligned with your beliefs. It's there to challenge you through your daily actions. Without my ego I would not be an Ironman. I have nurtured my ego to create the most magnificent results. Firstly, I listen and acknowledge that I have one, then embrace and respect it.

Getting started

Listen, acknowledge, breathe and use your power to move into action. Visualize guiding yourself through this process.

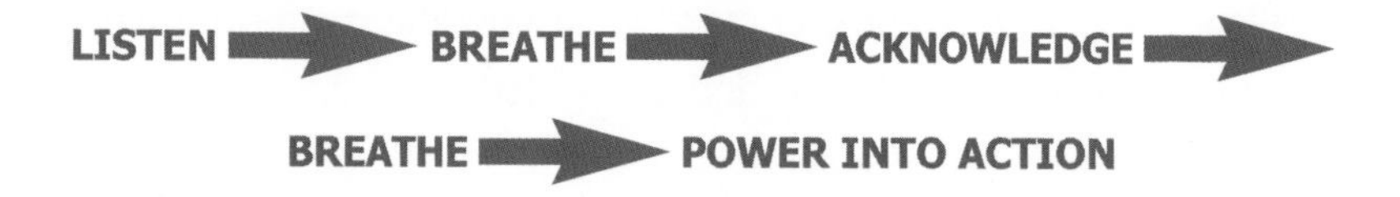

This is where you begin to journal your journey. It is a must for you to know yourself.

I have a powerful desire to share with you all that I know, the knowledge I have found on my lifelong journey to the extraordinary. You may laugh, but that is my mountain top. I'm not just dreaming big. I dream of gigantic shifts for women.

My purpose has evolved as my business has evolved. I find myself wanting to share and give more every day. This is why I loved nursing. These same values of sharing and giving complement my obsession with being my daily best.

My mission began with supporting people to move with purpose and ease. I can't help smiling just sharing with you now how that makes me feel: to empower people with the knowledge to create a better environment. Your environment starts with your body. Take care of your environment and disease cannot grow – or have I spelt 'disease' wrong? Dis-ease?

This spelling links to the concept of wellness in individuals and healing communities. Such a great thought!

My purpose has transformed into a breath-taking pitch. Every time I deliver my pitch, I allow it to land on people, watching their body language take the blow of such a power meaning.

I fell upon my purpose through my children. Their schools would set them homework, asking who their inspirations were. Louis, my little one, chose me as his life inspiration. How amazing is that? The feeling his words created in me have caused my greatest life changes. I was not aware of the impact I had made upon my children. I never celebrated my small wins. I didn't even acknowledge them. I lived in ignorance. Ignorance is never bliss.

Their image of me gave me an almighty push, an emotional push to honour my children's thoughts and the methodology I live by.

I knew from their innocent words that something significant was unfolding. They gave me my lifelong daily purpose, especially my daughter. She is a young, beautiful (inside and out), and powerful woman, and this prompted my biggest 'Why?'. Why didn't she seek the external world of fakery and forgeries, and the corrupt world of fashion and flawed role models? Happily, she looked closer to home; to her mumma.

My purpose, my waking thought, my daily vision, is for women to be their children's inspiration. The power of the word 'inspiration' excites me.

All that I know, I give: I am truly blessed to share and support you.

Birdonabike Is Born

'All it takes is faith, trust and pixie dust.'

Peter Pan

I knew I needed to find my purpose; it didn't even need to be mine, just any purpose. Ah, the concept of being needed. Everyone needs to be needed. I knew I was needed by my children and husband for the basics, but despite being responsible for the day-to-day running of a household I didn't feel needed. I felt I wasn't needed by anyone.

I did know that I needed to find a purpose., And I knew I had so much to give. But what? It's not easy searching for a purpose so I looked within, asking myself

- What do I love?
- What am I passionate about?
- What can I share with people that would make an impact on their lives?

ACTION

Ask yourself these same three questions and give yourself 5 minutes to find the answers from within your thoughts. Write your thoughts down in your journal and date this entry. When you return to these questions, your thoughts will create an instant smile as you recognize who you were at that moment.

I loved teaching. I had a thirst for knowledge. I loved fitness – some called it an obsession, but I would reply, 'What an awesome topic to be obsessed with!'.

Fitness is a basic human need for me, like breathing. It feeds my soul, it supports my mind and it builds my body. It is not something for which I take time out of my daily activities. No matter what I have in my schedule, fitness is part of my daily, weekly, monthly and annual schedule. Fitness is my priority. I never say I don't have or can't find enough time for fitness; time is something you cannot make or find. We all have the same 24 hours each day: the difference is that I always prioritise fitness.

I recognized my purpose: to teach people to move. To teach people to fall in love with fitness and lead them into a lifelong journey of health. I have always seen fitness as an investment in your future, and I wanted to share this concept with everyone I met.

I became a fitness instructor, then progressed into teaching Pilates, and progressed naturally into becoming a personal trainer. Personal training does not do justice to the knowledge I share with clients.

I respect you uniquely for being present in the moment of moving physically, whatever level you are at. I love seeing people of all shapes and sizes come into a class. Even if others judge you for not giving your best, I couldn't disagree more. Thank goodness people move from their homes to the gym, or go for a walk; thank goodness they move rather than sit at home with no oomph, watching TV, eating, hating – even loathing – themselves as they take each mouthful of food.

My initial mission became to support people to invest in their future health and movement. After endless searching and thought, how this has evolved!

The power of the word

I use language deliberately. I choose the structure and placement of words in my sentences carefully. The power of the word is strong. You often hear people say, 'Be careful with your words' or 'Choose your words wisely'. This is so true. Please become careful with your words.

Words create emotion, and emotion creates the momentum to action.

My gift to you: be kind to yourself. You are the one person you spend most of your time with. You are with yourself all day, so choose beautiful words for your internal dialogue. Your internal dialogue is the little chats you have with yourself throughout the day. Be mindful of your words, for your words know not what they do.

I am blessed to teach people to move with ease and purpose. To be able to help athletes reduce the risk of injury and speed recovery time is truly a dream come true. I love going into the homes of people who have minimal movement or ill health and support them to become strong and move around their environment more freely.

I want to share with you the stories of real people, so that they may create that final surge of energy or emotion for your 'had enough' moment to arrive. In each of these moments, the true human spirit jumps out of the page and into your being. Your emotions will be ignited and sparks will fly. Read with joy and a smile on your face.

Bill's 'had enough' moment

My skills and knowledge were challenged on meeting Bill. He wasn't my normal client – a busy mum wanting a body transformation or a competitive athlete. Bill's health wasn't good, but he wanted to move around his home more freely. Bill's wife, who had been attending Pilates with me for seven years, asked me for help – maybe I should call this Sue's 'had enough' moment, as Sue was desperately worried about her husband's health.

Bill wrote me a detailed letter explaining his medication and his past medical history. He explained his concerns about his present and future health. He was reaching out for support, but had no idea what help he needed. He was desperate to move freely.

Bill had given up smoking a year before he contacted me. He had been an active, strong, formidable character, but soon after his retirement his health deteriorated. He believed it was connected to stopping smoking. He could not leave the house because of a bowel problem, his mobility had reduced, and his spirit and mindset were weak. His desperation leapt out of the letter.

On my initial assessment with Bill, it was clear that simple mobility and body awareness were needed, developed through a respectful and informed approach. He gave me the greatest goal/gift I'd had from any other client to date. He touched my soul with these words: 'I want to be able to walk down to the bottom of my garden and back.'

The simplicity of this request struck my heart. To this day, I quote Bill's story, because it changed my understanding of fitness forever. I have felt pride in training amazing competitive athletes, from marathon to Iron Man level, where extreme levels of strength, commitment and courage are needed. We take it for granted that we can walk around our homes, but the goal Bill had identified was going to need all the strength, commitment and courage of an Iron Man.

For most people, health is the hat on a well person's head that only an ill person can see. How true this metaphor is. We only appreciate health when we don't have it.

I put together an achievable training plan, making Bill's home his gym. The programme was a 12-week gentle mobility and strengthening course to build Bill's confidence, awareness and understanding of his body's capabilities. I gave him functional exercises for homework: sitting on an upright stool, maintaining good posture, alternating leg lifts, all while having a cup of tea with his wife.

Bill thrived not just on the exercises but on interaction with a human being other than his wonderful wife. While Bill trained, Sue was given the gift of time, to catch up on simple household jobs. Just filling in forms in peace and quiet was uplifting for her.

Halfway through Bill's programme, I started to focus him on his next mountain top achievement: going on holiday.

The great day came. Bill had not only nailed walking down to the bottom of his garden and back, but also down his driveway. There was no stopping him; he was now going out for walks with his wife, gently, safely and with glowing pride in his achievements.

Bill continues on his journey of health and movement. During his 12-week programme it became apparent that Bill has the most wonderful gift of storytelling. Not only does he relay his historical stories with a tone of anarchy and wit, but he is also able to translate this into the written word. With some encouragement and confidence-building, Bill is now writing his life story in weekly chapters.

Book trail

Bernstein, G. (2014). *May Cause Miracles: A 40-day guidebook of subtle shifts for radical change and unlimited happiness.* New York: Harmony. (Kindle edition available)

Johnson, S. (1998). *Who Moved My Cheese? An amazing way to deal with change in your work and your life.* London: Simon and Schuster. (Kindle edition available)

Pransky, J. (2011). *Somebody Should Have Told Us: Simple truths for living well. CCB Publishers.* (Kindle edition available)

Sharma, R. (2010). *The Leader Who Had No Title: A modern fable on real success in business and in life.* London: Vermilion.

Vitale, J. and Hibbler, B. (2006). *Meet and Grow Rich: How to easily create and operate your own mastermind group health, wealth, and more.* New York: John Wiley & Sons. (Kindle edition available)

2

Your Thoughts

'Any day spent with you is my favourite day. So, today is my new favourite day.'

Winnie the Pooh

For 20 years, I believed that you must have physical health before building your focus and mindset. But I would not be being true to you or myself if I had kept to this limiting belief. Health must also come from within before you add stress to your body by using exercise to build a strong framework. Your internal dialogue needs you to listen to it, allow it to be heard. Once you are aware of the dialogue, then and only then, can adaptation begin.

Once you hear your internal chatter, you begin to understand yourself: how you cope in challenging day-to-day situations, what you resist in life, how you use distraction as a non-coping mechanism. Remember, I use my words deliberately: a non-coping mechanism.

A non-coping mechanism is you telling yourself you are dealing with a challenge when all you are doing is diverting yourself from the pain. How can you become a problem-solver, when you won't even acknowledge to yourself that there is one?

Distraction is my biggest non-coping mechanism. I'm the busiest person I know and I have the most energy. But my personal energy has massive peaks, and then drops from the greatest of heights. I had been doing this for years. I was exhausted.

I had to stop this destructive behaviour, so I listened to me. I became an observer of me, using self-time as a must. This created momentary pain. It's like hitting your elbow: it's excruciating to begin with, but it fades and you continue with your day. Once you've gone through this process, you will find longer periods of personal peace.

You will discover in Chapter 9 the magic of daily rituals. Within the daily rituals is self-time. Self-time will be your greatest gift to yourself. You will discover your beliefs and values, your passions and dreams, your long- and short-tern goals, how you feel and how you want to feel. Notice the word 'your':

- Are your beliefs and values yours?
- Are your dreams and passions yours?
- Are your goals or outcomes yours?

If you have not invested in self-time, where you find out about you, my guess is that they're not. I'm not suggesting that I know you, but I know human behaviour; I've studied behaviour, why we do what we do, our movements, the rituals of the time- poor, and why and how humans can change their behaviour.

Our values and beliefs are usually handed down to us from our parents' parents' parents, or maybe from even further back along our ancestry. Realizing this was a massive tipping point for me. Firstly, I held a strong belief system, but on reflection realized that much of it didn't belong to me. Secondly, if they weren't mine it was because they were out of date, not relevant to me now. You could call this my revelation.

ACTION

Take 5 minutes to create self-time space in your day to discover your thoughts, to examine these elements:

- Your beliefs and values
- Your passion and dreams
- Your long- and short-term goals
- Write your thoughts in your journal.

Writing down thoughts and ideas bears witness to the moment of those feelings. It makes them a real commodity, not just thoughts in the ether. Writing neatly with pen and paper imprints them in your nervous system more efficiently than if you use a computer. It stimulates and fine-tunes the health of your motor skills. Daily practice demonstrates your commitment.

Relax into your findings. They may cause you some agitation. Relax into your feelings, into the present moment. The less frantic you are about these findings, the more space it creates to adapt.

Malcolm Gladwell describes this moment as the 'tipping point'. The feelings you are observing, the answers you are exploring will give clarity. This in turn creates momentum and here is your tipping point. Momentum is movement; the visual of something tipping over the edge allows us to see movement in action.

The tipping point is subjective: it relates only to you and your experiences, for one person's tipping point is another's coping point. You can't make comparisons or judgments. This point tips you into your 'had enough' moment'.

You just haven't had enough

Have you ever got to that point where you think you can't take any more? Are 'I have had enough' or 'I can't take any more' familiar words, whether concerning relationships, the behaviour of others towards you, or your own internal happiness? Body image is one of the most frequent causes of women's 'had enough' moments: too fat, too wobbly – they hate themselves. Women grab the parts they hate and shake them with disdain, pointing angrily at them. Strong words, but true.

Nicola's 'had enough' moment

A super-confident lady (well, that's what the outside world would see), oozing with personality, came to me with these words: 'I hate my jelly belly, I have great legs, I love my boobs, but I loathe my tummy.'

Nicola had two children, ten years apart. She was 37 years old, with beautiful skin, super pretty, the kind of lady you want to poke in the eyes (joking, of course). Nicola was uber-stylish; she could make a bin bag look so amazing you'd probably even ask her 'where did you get your dress from?' Very French-looking.

But she was right: her tummy was an untoned mass, giving her a barrel effect. Her clothes did not fit; she felt unattractive in clothes and out of them, and periodically rejected her fiancé's advances. She refused to get undressed in front of him, but had tried the underwear trick. (What's the underwear trick? Wearing nice underwear makes you feel good, even when you're at the supermarket. Even bigger tip for the underwear trick: it must be matching.) But this was still failing her.

Nicola carried these feelings of self-loathing, of disgust, of fatness around all day, every day. She dreaded the school playground, feeling she was being glared at and ridiculed for losing her shape. We humans find beauty in others a personal threat. It can create feelings of jealousy, but I believe it can even create fear in us: fear of our partners moving towards the beauty they perceive in another person. She felt everybody loved her getting fat; she said she had had enough, and with desperation asked for my support.

Does Nicola's story sound familiar to you? What's your 'had enough'? This is a great time to reflect on this question that will be the beginning of an incredible personal journey towards greatness.

ACTION

Take a timer and time 2 minutes. Just be. Ask yourself 'Have I had enough?'

Have you thought you have had enough but somehow carried on with your day, your routines, and your life without changing or adapting your behaviour?

Write down anything and everything that comes into your mind. Do not edit, let the words flow. Physically write in your notebook. I always buy a lovely journal-type notepad, A5 size so that I can fit it in my bag to take everywhere with me. Odd moments pop up during the day when, if you don't take it with you, you will wish you had. Get into the habit. Sometimes days just don't go the way you have planned. This makes the most of the hours in my day. Thoughts and feelings come at the weirdest of times.

I have just been introduced to the Dictaphone on my mobile. I felt so awkward to start with, but if I can do it with a gruff, squeaky Devonshire accent, then anyone can. Just talk into it. Say everything and anything. Allow pauses. Just get it out there. It's OK to feel your emotions take shape. It does get easier. I confided to my friend Stephanie about the power of the Dictaphone, and my fear of using this function that has apparently been on my mobile forever. We both agreed that after a while we enjoyed listening back to our voices.

Book trail

Ariely, D. (2009). *Predictably Irrational: The hidden forces that shape our decisions.* London: HarperCollins. (Kindle edition available)

Ben-Shahar, T. (2007). *Happier: Learn the secrets to daily joy and lasting fulfilment.* Maryland: HighBridge. (Audiobook)

Dalai Lama, The and Cutler, H.C.(1999). *The Art of Happiness: A handbook for living.* London: Hodder & Stoughton. (Kindle edition available)

Gandhi, M.K. and Khilnani, S (2001). *An Autobiography: The story of my experiments with the truth.* London: Penguin. (Kindle edition available)

Gladwell, M., Ross, L. and Nisbett, R.E. (2011). *The Person and the Situation: Perspectives of social psychology*. London: Pinter & Martin. (Kindle edition available)

Polis, B. (2006). *Only a Mother Could Love Him*. London: Hodder & Stoughton.

Pressfield, S. (2012). *The War of Art: Break through the blocks and win your inner creative battles*. Black Irish Entertainment LLC. (Kindle edition available)

Pressfield, S. (2012). *Turning Pro: Tap you inner power and create your life's work*. Black Irish Entertainment LLC. (Kindle edition available)

3

Your Feelings

'Close your eyes. Now forget what you see.
What do you feel?'
Tarzan

What are your feelings? How do you feel at this moment? This question to myself started as, 'How do I feel today?' but I became aware that this was too generic. Throughout my day my feelings would change, not just emotional ones but physical ones, too, depending on my training and the intensity of my daily plan.

So ask yourself the greatest question, 'How do I feel at this moment?'

This is a beautiful gift to give yourself: asking yourself and listening to the feedback. Ask yourself this question throughout the day. It's fascinating what you hear.

This practice goes deeper. What are feelings? Where do you feel things and how does that feel in the body? Feelings are thoughts manifested within you, moving from the mind into your physical cellular structure. Thoughts are actioned into the cells to create feelings, which in turn create human behaviour. By analyzing your thoughts, with the help of the Dictaphone or your daily journal entries, you can understand why you feel and behave as you do. But if you never allow yourself the time, you remain in ignorance of yourself, behaving like a robot, programmed, lifeless, moving unconsciously.

Please remember: ignorance is never bliss.

My gift to you is to get you asking yourself great questions. The challenge now is knowing what is a great question is. It's personal. Asking yourself how you feel about things is good place to start. To become aware of your feelings, or of how you want to feel, is exciting.

Committing to a goal or outcome provides a great opportunity to focus on your feelings. I love racing: marathons, Iron Man, duathlons. I love the idea of completing such an achievement. You don't have to choose such extreme or endurance sports. Just committing to train to your goal is an extraordinary act. But along the journey of training, how do you want to feel? I want to enjoy each day of training. I want to feel strong within my body and spirit. I want to laugh and have fun with my training buddies. It's not just about achieving your goal and then waiting to see how that makes you feel. It's about each moment along the way.

The lessons and skills I learned and put into practice in training and sport are transferrable to any circumstance in life.

My gift to you is: ask yourself, what are your centred feelings? What desires do you have? What feelings does this create in your centre, your core? What is your gut feeling, your intuition?

ACTION

Take five minutes to write in your journal.

Note down your answers to these questions:

- What feelings do I want to create every day?
- What will it look and feel like to have those feelings?

These feelings, once identified, are super-powerful. They are interchangeable. You don't have to keep them. Be playful. Know that at any time you can choose more suitable feelings for the moment you find yourself in.
Mine at the moment are: Wise, Strong, Fun and Grateful.

I want to be wise. I want to use my wisdom.
I want to be strong in my thoughts, in my physiology, and in my spiritual existence.
I want to have, and be, fun, every day of every year.
I want to always be grateful for the world around me, for the breath I take.

Each day, at each moment, I think, how do I want to feel about this?
I fail at this sometimes. But I work on my emotional muscle continuously. This is self-love.

ACTION

Take 5 minutes

During your daily ritual of reflection, ask yourself:
What are my daily desired feelings?
Choose between two and six – having too many may create resistance.
Write them in your journal and why you want to feel that way.
Review them monthly as life evolves and they change. You may not need to change them. You may love them so much they are lifelong feelings.

Now you have discovered how you want to feel along the journey, you can start to shape your vision, your aspirations, your own mountain top.

Visualising

Visualizing is a powerful tool. The ability to see what is not there or to imagine the impossible is what makes humans extraordinary. Visualizing is most commonly used in sport. Sir Roger Bannister was renowned for this practice. The 4-minute mile had never been achieved – over thousands of years, no one had never run that fast. It was suggested that humans had reached their land speed limit in regard to land speed. But in 1954 one man smashed that belief by running 1 mile in 3 minutes 59.4 seconds.

We still use his training methods of training today: interval, anaerobic, periodisation and fell-running. But his ability to believe and to see what was not there was also a skill he mastered. Interestingly, once he had broken the record, it only took 46 days for it to be broken again. Bannister had made the impossible possible.

His quotes are inspirational:

'The man who can drive himself further once the effort gets painful is the man who will win.'

This illustrates the journey you have started on. It will not be easy: there will be challenges, it will get painful, but go through the pain and victory will prevail.

Keep moving forward.

Book trail

Allen, J. (2013). *As a Man Thinketh.* CreateSpace Independent Publishing Platform. (Kindle edition available)

Kramer, G. (2012). *Stillpower: Excellence with ease in sports and life.* Hillsboro: Beyond Words Publishing. (Kindle edition available)

Rath, T. (2007). *Strengths Finder 2.0.* Gallup Press. (Kindle edition available)

Ruiz, D.M. Jnr (2013). *The Five Levels of Attachment.* San Antonio: Hierophant Publishing. (Kindle edition available)

Wattles, W. D. and Legins, A.W. (2013). The Science of Getting Rich for Women! CreateSpace Independent Publishing Platform.

4

Mastering Focus

'What you think you become. What you feel you attract. What you imagine you create.'

Buddha

Focus means channeling your thoughts, cultivating feelings and taking action to support your feelings. This process creates an abundance of energy at the start, but it requires discipline to maintain your vision – the art of remaining focused.

Self-time should have given you the momentum to develop and master the skill of focus. Focus starts with your thoughts, your wonderful ideas and your innermost dreams, creating an energy, a cellular vibration causing excitement and a 'behind-the-eyes' story.

Again, a great place to start is to ask great questions.

1. Where am I now? Give a real and honest account of your present thoughts.
2. Where do I want to be? Start with the end in mind. Focus your thought on your destination.
3. How do I get there? What tools can assist me in my journey towards my destination. What resources do I need?

I have recently applied these questions to building my own focus skills. I had a bike accident a year ago, and I am lucky I can still move, let alone run. The accident meant I could not rush around being busy all day long. I was in excruciating pain and had limited mobility. I didn't have the distraction of clients or friends. I had to spend time with me! It was 'interesting'.

I use the word with a slight curl of my lip. At first pain relief provided a marvelous distortion of my thoughts and then television did likewise. But there are only so many movies and serials one human can cope with watching.

I had studied the habits and thoughts of the most successful people on the planet for years, and I knew that self-discovery would take me into a new chapter of my journey towards being true to myself. I set aside small chunks of allocated time within my day to drown myself in self-time. When I say 'small chunks', I mean one minute per day of sitting with my thoughts, then recording the findings. This started as a painful process, but with each passing day, I added one minute to the total time. Very quickly this one-minute chunk of time grew to five minutes, then, within a month, I was bathing in my thoughts of love and creativity for 30 minutes at a time. No more drowning. It was a beautiful place to be. My favourite time of day for self-time is in the magic hour between 5 a.m. and 6a.m. Its stillness brings an excitement to the waiting day.

ACTION

Creating to the power of five

Find a space that you dedicate to this practice, which takes only 5 minutes of self-time. This is essential for the process to take hold. Remember, you are building new pathways of behaviour. Using the same space engages the brain, allowing it to predict how it should behave – just as you know when you go to the shower room what is going to happen. This phenomenon is discussed in Chapter 6, Neuroplasticity.

- Write in your journal, recording the date and time. Breathe.
- Write the names of five support networks around you. Breathe
- Write five things you want to achieve in your life. Breathe
- Write five things that describe where you are now in your life. Breathe
- Sit and reflect for 2 minutes. Try not to read or go over what you have just written.

Smile and congratulate yourself. You have completed a challenging stage of the process. Little wins, little wins, little wins create one quantum leap.

What did you discover about yourself? Did you enjoy the time to breathe? Did you feel comfortable within yourself? How did you feel about answering the questions?

Taking self-time, answering great questions, produces great answers. This simple yet effective stage enables you to clarify your thoughts, feelings, wants and needs. With clarity comes power. The feeling of power within creates cellular vibrations. A cell vibrating is pure energy being built from within your physiology.

You do not have an organic abundance of energy; you you create your own personal energy.

I believe that no matter how tired or fatigued I am, if I focus on creating momentum then I become super-energized. Energy is movement. Motion is created from emotion. You have brought your emotions, feelings, and thoughts to life. Your focus has generated clear outcomes. Your clarity brought together with your focus has a nuclear impact upon your personal energy. When we have clarity, power and energy, the momentum is unstoppable. And you have generated all of this within five minutes.

You Are Amazing. Did you see, did you hear, and did you accept these beautiful words? My gift to you.

My best friend compliments me all the time. I find it a challenge, to say the least. I don't see what he sees in me, but he shared his wisdom: 'Accept compliments, as they are not given freely or frequently.' The more we throw back at the wonderful giving person, the less we will receive. It is a gift; accept it – even if it is through gritted teeth.

To develop this practice, write the 'powerful five' from your journal on A3 paper. Put it on your wall; make it real. I love it. It keeps you focused from the minute you wake up. I have about three A3 sheets on my bedroom wall: my 'powerful fives', my dreams and passions, and a portrait of my ideal client. (There is a very funny story behind this drawing: my eldest is an amazing artist. When I asked him to draw my ideal client, describing what she would look like, it looked like a rock and roll star.) I now have a beautiful magazine picture of what my client looks like which I have personalized by sticking it to A3 and writing her characteristics around the picture. Everyday I see her, her eyes, her pain, what she wants and how I can support. Everyday I breath her in.

I don't know about you, but I have ideas and thoughts flooding my mind hourly. Yet I sometimes talk myself out of what I want, coming off the path of my journey. When you lose focus it's challenging to return to your pathway, and it wastes energy. This simple, effective, drawing is there when I wake, it's in my day, and now in my dreams.

Your dreams, your visions build your subconscious.

Book trail

Alexander, S. (2003). *Rhinoceros Success: The secret to charging full speed towards every opportunity*. Ramsey Solutions Inc. (Kindle edition available)

Clason, G. S. (2015). *The Richest Man in Babylon*. New York: Signet. (Kindle edition available). First published in 1926.

Dispenza, J. (2009). *Evolve Your Brain: The science of changing your mind*. Deerfield Beach, FLA: Health Communications Inc. (Kindle edition available)

Irvine, B. (2012). *Einstein and the Art of Mindful Cycling: Achieving balance in the modern world*. Lewes: Ivy Press.

Shinn, F.S. (2010). *The Complete Works*. New York: Dover Publications Inc. (Kindle edition available) First published in 1940.

5

Manifesting Your Mindset

'No matter how your heart is grieving, if you keep on believing, the dream that you wish will come true.'

Cinderella

A mindset is the ideas and attitudes through which a person approaches a certain situation, especially when they are difficult to change.

Carol Dweck is one of the world's leading researchers in the field of motivation. She focuses on why people succeed, and she categorizes mindsets as 'fixed' or 'growth'. We more commonly call mindsets positive or negative. Having a positive mindset/attitude allows your success to grow, hence a 'growth' mindset. Having a negative mindset/attitude allows no scope for adaptation and therefore it is a 'fixed' mindset. Your mindset determines failure or success. To have a positive or growth mindset is instrumental to achieving your goals.

Dr Norman Vincent Peale, author of *The Power of Positive Thinking*, said,

'Formulate and stamp indelibly on your mind a mental picture of yourself as succeeding. Hold this picture tenaciously and never permit it to fade. Your mind will seek to develop this picture!' Positive thinking gives space for creativity to grow. Allowing the mind to build images of success can only come from thinking positively. You'll hear me say this time and time again: 'It's simple but it's not easy.'

(You will be finishing my sentences for me as we go through this journey together, like an old married couple.)

Benjamin Disraeli, former British Prime Minister and statesman said, 'Nurture your mind with great thoughts, for you will never go any higher than you think.'

This is such a powerful statement. Allow these words to sink into your mind. Allow your thoughts to absorb them and your feelings to understand them.

Your thoughts are your internal dialogue within your mindset. You are the master of your thoughts. You choose what you chat to yourself about. Do we have a choice of what we think and feel? Do we choose to be positive or negative in our mindset?

Why would anyone choose to think negatively about something?

Do we choose to believe in our dreams or listen to others tearing our dreams down around us? Even worse, do we listen to ourselves talking ourselves out of them?

These are not rhetorical questions. They should make you stop and analyze your everyday thoughts, feelings and actions. Why would we be unkind to ourselves, or allow others to be unkind to us?

Choice relies on the mental ability to make a decision. But what if you are not skilled in making decisions? What if you hate having a choice?

What if you hate making decisions? What if you feel you're not allowed to make decisions? Too many choices mean no decision. When we don't know which choice to make, we often decide to take neither option. Being aware of who we are, what skills we find challenging, and having strategies to embrace action can help us when we are stuck in this way.

But choice also implies opportunity. Choices create opportunities. This makes me smile. The only answer to all of the challenging questions I have posed is 'yes'. You always have a choice, even if you don't want to make one. We all have a choice. It might not be the choice we want, but nevertheless choice we have.

External strategies to create energy

A useful physical strategy to practise is your awareness posture. Putting your body into a position of alignment will create an internal power you have not felt before. You are balancing your internal energy, balancing your chakras. This may be your first introduction to chakras. They are explained in Chapter 9, in the section on Daily Ritual 7.

ACTION

The ABCs of awareness posture

- A – Alignment: in a seated position, align your posture, so that you feel balanced and peaceful.
- B – Breath: In your beautiful seated posture, breathe deep and wide into your ribcage. This practice is challenging, as naturally you will breathe into the upper part of your chest. Visualize breathing deep down into your abdomen, so that your rib-cage opens out to the sides, like an accordion, rather than moves up.
- C – Centre: centre your posture on your seat bones – the two prominent bones in your bottom. (There's no point in shouting 'I can't feel them, as my bum is too big,' at me; I'm not listening!) Engage your tummy muscles (abdominals); keep your ribcage active but not flaring – flaring of the ribcage encourages the back to bend like a banana. Keep the ribcage connected down towards the hips.

Use this action every time a decision is needed. I promise you it will generate great power. This posture is a trigger to your mind to behave in a certain way and it therefore creates the conditions for decision-making. The more frequently you use this technique the greater the skill you develop for creating powerful opportunities from daily choices.

Just say No

Begin to use the word **No** to protect your thoughts.
Begin to stay focused on your vision.

Begin to align your vision to opportunities that drop into your day.

Steve Jobs created a lifestyle that we find ourselves living today. He said, 'We're here to put a dent in the universe.' Take this one step further: being *you* is all about putting a dent in the universe. Each moment in his life brought countless opportunities and disappointments. He used the experience he gained from Pixar to reach his mountain top, and his vision now lives as his legacy.

In 1986, after he had been fired from the company he co-founded, Apple Mackintosh, Steve Jobs purchased a computer graphics division from George Lucas and established a company called Pixar. Pixar gave him the understanding of single focus through *Toy Story*. Pixar's ethos was to concentrate on one product, becoming obsessed with it to the exclusion of everything else. Focus on one extraordinary thing and do it really, really well. Become Pixar.

Steve Jobs returned to Apple and used this focus in one area of the business. He found that their vision was diluted across a vast number of products. He focused Apple's vision on the iPod and look what happened.

Confucius supposedly said, 'The man who chases two rabbits, catches neither.' Focus on one thing that will take you to the next level of your journey to your mountain top. Saying no protects your energy, protects you from spreading yourself too thin, from people wanting more of you, all of which could dilute your ideas. Such power comes when you say 'No!' aloud. You need to remain open to the many opportunities that come your way in life. Begin to recognize opportunities that are aligned with your mountain top: opportunities are only opportunities if they serve you.

Many opportunities will come; they can make you feel amazing, but choose them wisely, with clarity and focus, to ensure they are aligned with your vision. Be aware that others may see them as opportunities for themselves, but need you to support their goals.

You are on a quest, a quest to create your vision, your mountain top adventure. The universe will challenge you. You may fail at times – no, you will fail many times. This is part of the process of success, so have the courage to say 'no' when you need to. Only you know what is right for you.

The word 'courage' originates from an Old French word from around 1300: 'corage', meaning 'heart, innermost feelings'. When you come from a place of love for yourself, then you are able to decide whether this is an opportunity that you should take. Using courage to say no to opportunities means that you are coming from your innermost feelings for what is right for you.

Here's a wonderful way of listening to your internal intentions.

The 60-second rule

Known in business as the 90-second rule, we can refine it to do the same in 60 seconds. This method shrinks your mental deadline, an idea reflected in Parkinson's Law: 'work expands to fill the time available'.

ACTION

Applying the 60-second rule

When an opportunity or an idea comes up, apply the 60-second rule, and take the following steps for saying 'No' if that is what you need to do.

Let the opportunity or idea land on you.

- Take 60 seconds to focus only on the opportunity/thought at that moment.
- Stay in the moment.
- Filter distractions, strip away the noise.
- Edit the idea/opportunity, simplify its application.
- Make the decision, always moving it forward.

Jack's 'had enough' moment'

Paralyzed with the fear of making the wrong decision, Jack lives by the belief that he is unable to make decisions. He feels unable to cope with any change, positive or negative. He knows how to behave where he is right now. If change happens, which of course is the only thing in life that we can guarantee, how should he behave?

Jack was leaving college, where he excelled. You would think he would have been full of confidence, but no. He had a passion but began to question whether he truly wanted to go along his chosen pathway.

The most important element for Jack was that he didn't want to feel like this anymore. He had reached his 'had enough' moment. He was petrified of the future but had a total understanding that things couldn't stay the same. He had a vision, but lacked unwavering faith. In fact, he had little to no faith in his vision or ability to act.

I supported Jack to re-evaluate his vision, his passion. Did he really still love and want to continue on this pathway? The answer was 'yes'.

Now began the process of allowing Jack to see just how amazing he was. Getting him to make a decision gave him momentum, forward movement brought emotion to his decision. His confidence grew quickly. Small decisions and little tweaks to the language Jack used on a daily basis, permitted him to make more and bigger decisions. For Jack, the future had created such fear it stopped him in his tracks.

Bringing the future closer creates momentum in daily decisions and activates the skill of decision-making. As Al Pacino said, 'Life is a game of inches'.

The inch you achieve today builds towards the mile you walk next week. Take small steps towards what you want, moving forward one step every day. These steps will eventually amount to a quantum leap into your vision.

Stay courageous and dance with fear.
Stay calm.
Stay consistent.

Book trail

Heath, C. and D. (2013). *Decisive: How to make better choices in life and work.* New York: Random House Business. (Kindle edition available.)

Hill, N. (2007). The Magic Ladder to Success. New York: Jeremy P. Tarcher. (Kindle edition available) First published in 1930.

Maslow, A. H. (1983). Religions: Values and Peak-Experiences. Gloucester, Mass., Peter Smith Publishers. (Kindle edition available)

Maslow, A. H. (2014). *Toward a Psychology of Being.* Bensenville, Ill.: Lushena Books. (Kindle edition available)

Sapolsky, R. (2004). *Why Zebras Don't Get Ulcers.* New York: St Martin's Press.

6

Neuroplasticity – The Art of Learning New Habits

'The flower that blossoms in adversity is the most rare and beautiful of them all'

The Emperor, *Mulan*

This chapter introduces you to how humans learn. What different theories and opinions are there about creating and adapting daily habits? For me, the answer is simple: ask yourself the greatest questions every day, and focus on the answers, the action you need to take, and implement the tweaks consistently.

I have found that using the word 'change' creates negative, challenging thoughts and behaviour in people. The word 'tweaks' creates a smile, an element of fun. It generates a will to action, not a spirit of resistance.

I have studied the world's leading authorities on human behaviour, on why we do what we do. It fascinates me. Knowledge alone is not the answer, but it is the beginning.

The brain is able to adapt itself by forming new neural connections throughout your life. *Encyclopedia Britannica* states that learning reflects the capacity of neurons (nerve cells) and their networks in the brain to alter their connections and behaviour in response to new information, sensory stimulation, development, damage or dysfunction.

Neuroplasticity is the brain's ability to reorganize itself by building new pathways, creating a new infrastructure within the brain. This is also called brain plasticity or brain malleability.

How long does it take to form a new habit? Some research indicates that if you practise a new behaviour for 6 weeks – that's 180 days – you will begin to rewire your neural system. I have been researching how to form new habits and how long this process takes, at length. I have found conflicting views, ranging from 21 days to 254 days. Don't react – breathe, we are all different. Let me help you put some sense into the vast amount of conflicting evidence.

The most recent piece of research looks at the 21-day habit myth. This came from Dr Maxwell Maltz, a plastic surgeon psychologist, who studied recovering facelift patients. He suggested in 1960 that it takes a patient 21 days to get used to his/her new face. We have taken this specific anecdotal evidence and generalized it to include the completely different activity of incorporating a new habit into your daily routine.

A study in 2010 carried out more vigorous research into habit formation. This study of health-promoting behaviour tracked participants over 84 days. The researchers saw a large difference between individuals' ability to reach their peak practice, ranging from 18 days to 254 days. The research concluded that 66 days was the average length of time it took for a new habit to form.

So, let me bring all of this relevant information together. Some of the top global coaches state that it takes 66 days to form new habits. Robin Sharma has recently released online information confirming this, using the terminology of neuroplasticity.

Neuroplasticity is an umbrella term for the brain's ability to make lifelong changes. 'Neuro' meaning nerve cells in our brain; 'plastic' meaning pliable, flexible and easy to mold.

Dr Michael Merzenich, world renowned neuroscientist, explains the importance of neuroplasticity:

'My brain power depends on my retained mastery of analyzing in detail what's happening in my world and in my mind and body. I must continue to practise to retain my constructive and analytic powers. The goal is to be a master of my environment.'

Mastering your environment is an essential element of implementing new behaviour.

I have created a program based upon the latest research combining neuroplasticity and the time factor to cement new life habits. The results are astounding. This time span gives you personal momentum for lifelong behavioural change.

Debbie's 'had enough' moment

Busy being busy being busy.

Debbie was actually proud of being busy, telling me she loved being busy, buzzing around getting everything done. But... every day she woke up fatigued. Every day, as her eyes opened, she waited for the dreaded feeling of exhaustion. Every day, she waited for her body to ache from every cell.

Every day, knowing that even the unconscious movement of breathing hurt, she wanted it to stop.

Every day, she wanted... what? She didn't even have the energy to think.

Debbie was a super successful single-mum and high achieving businesswoman, but felt every day that she had nothing left to give. She loathed this feeling, but loved her children and was proud of her business – well, intermittently.

She had massive peaks and troughs of energy throughout the day, spiking at 11:00 in the morning and dropping like a stone at 15:30 just as her family needed her energy and love. She believed in good food, regular visits to the gym, but knew that she had reached her 'had enough' moment.

She came to me at this critical point. She acknowledged her amazing achievements but she wanted to feel love again and more energy throughout the day, not crash and burn at 15:30 after picking up her little one and getting home. Home did not bring peace.

Debbie was super-tired when she got home and protective of her time, making her very impatient and reluctant to do anything with the little ones after supper. Life was definitely not as she had imagined it would be two years after her divorce. Her finances were manageable, but only just, and she missed the family life that once was. How do you move forward when you are paralyzed in the past and have no energy to give to the future?

Debbie saw an online interview with me. She was drawn to my energy and understanding of 'what women want'. She loved the idea of me championing women, and she was desperate to be an inspiration to her children.

The 66-Day Programme sent Debbie into a whirl. It was not what she expected at all. Her preconceptions dominated the first five days, and she would ask, 'What is all this about?' Her resistance had immediately raised its ugly head.

But on the weekly Q&A drop-ins I noticed Debbie was overcoming this. She began to participate in her own life; allocating a time to read her emails and action them became a daily ritual for her.

No more loving the feeling of being busy being busy being busy.
No more spikes of energy and lows of emotion.
No more loathing the life she led.
No more hating her beautiful body.

Having a love for the life she was creating made a huge impact on her children. She engaged with them on their return from school, wanting to hear their daily adventures. Having the energy and the willpower to go on days out, she inspired her children to become masters at making 'Magic Moments'.

Debbie's vision appeared. She was able to see her children's smiles, to hear the fun through laughter and to feel love and warmth through hugs.

Participation in the daily rituals gave Debbie the feelings she desired, every day. Actioning daily consistent rituals or habits began the process of creating the life Debbie desired. She now has unwavering faith from within, unwavering faith in her abilities to be her children's inspiration.

Learning is simple but not easy

A healthy brain is hungry to learn throughout life, although we have an in-built resistance to change. How many times have you heard the phrase 'I don't like change'? My son Jack has adapted this phrase to 'I don't do change'. Either way, this phrase blocks the capacity to learn.

Resistance to change is healthy. It's part of being human, but when we resist out of fear, it blocks development and inhibits progress. Fear arises from our beliefs and what we perceive to be true. This is a 'hunter-gatherer' protection or defence. It is primal, imprinted in the memory cells of our body. The body releases stress hormones to protect itself from pain or discomfort, so in effect learning is inhibited hormonally (although there is an opposing view that stress sometimes enhances the ability to learn.)

As humans we are simple beings. We react to stimuli with either pain or pleasure. If there is a choice between pleasure and pain, the decision is obvious: pleasure wins. But if it is between two pain stimuli, the lesser of the pains wins.

ACTION

Gain from your pain

Take five minutes to consider what your pains are.

What would be two pains that you could consciously choose between, and which is the lesser? Write your thoughts and feelings in your journal and date them.

This is a discovery exercise. No answers to be found yet. Merely to understand what your thoughts are and to make them visible to you.

Take food as an example. I dislike offal with a vengeance. Liver or kidneys? Both are pain stimuli to me, even though I can apply logic to this dilemma. Although I have a deep knowledge of nutrition and I know that offal is a super-food for our bodies, I still have the problem that this is a choice between two pain stimuli.

Being aware of who you are, of what your pleasure and pain triggers are, gives you control over the fear that is a natural protective response.

Our brain makes decisions on whether to accept new learning or specific change. Learning therefore requires new ways of thinking. Neuroplasticity.

Implementing new learning can be laborious and overwhelming. It takes an immense amount of work, emotion and time.

Most new behaviour or changes to acquired, formed behavior occur in the subconscious mind. Specific action is needed to allow the conscious mind to imprint behaviour change on the unconscious mind.

There are three stages in new learning:

1. Awareness and an understanding of our fears and stressors. We may want to learn new information or skills, but we don't always want to embrace the learning process. In other words, we might have a tantrum when we have to work at a project, and evade the task in hand – doing anything physically possible other than getting on with the task, housework or writing that essay.
2. Thinking patterns within our activities of daily living (ADLs – your daily routine). 'I don't have time to learn a new skill', 'I'm already busy and overloaded'. Sound familiar?
3. When you action new behaviour, challenging the fear, energy flows. You start off with excitement at the prospect of a bright future; it often becomes a bit sticky in the middle, but then the fog lifts and it all becomes clear. It's a roller coaster of emotions.

What does all this mean? It means that old dogs can learn new tricks. A great analogy for this is a tall-growing wheat field. A narrow pathway has been trodden down by walkers. It would be less effort to go along this path, but you might find it doesn't take you to where you want to go. As humans, we always take the path of least resistance.

Taking a pathway that hasn't been trodden by anyone else is heading into the unknown. You know the end result you want, but the route is unmarked. You make the first mark. It takes will, knowledge and determination to repeat this action, but over time the path becomes easier to travel as you adapt to the effort required. The repetition of traveling along the more efficient route changes your pathway. The same is true of neural pathways.

'Repetition is the mother of all skill.' Tony Robbins repeats this quote throughout his seminars. I have continued to use it when teaching: Repetition, Repetition, Repetition.

John Wooden, the legendary American basketball player and coach, said, 'The importance of repetition until automaticity cannot be overstated.' Repetition is the key to learning. Repeating a new behaviour, daily, even though you may fail, will result in success. Use this mantra: 'Repetition Repetition Repetition. Results Results Results.'

I'll make a cheerleader out of you yet!

Pareto's Principle: The 80-20 Rule

Also known as the Law of the Vital Few, this is based on the fact that for many events, 80% of the effects comes from 20% of the causes. The history of this principle comes from Italy, where economist Vilfredo Pareto observed in 1906 that 80% of the land was owned by 20% of the population. The 80-20 Rule is widely used throughout business, specifically in sales and marketing. It's an efficacy principle: the majority of results come from a minority of inputs.

Focus on the activities in your life that produce the best outcomes for you. You could transfer this to your ADLs: which are more productive? Use this principle if you find implementing new daily rituals overwhelms you. Review them and make a positive conscious decision on which ones have priority. Then implement 20% of them.

Effect change one tweak at a time. Assess which tweak will meet with the least resistance but give enormous gains – quick wins. Enjoy this process. Smile. These small tweaks will set you on fire. You will be bursting and vibrating with energy. I cannot emphasize enough how important awareness is. It is the key to change. This will give you momentum. By doing what you love more often you will find greater fulfillment.

Fake it till you make it

This was a new concept for me. It's not a method I thought I used in my business, but when I analyzed my business style, I realise that I do use this style to my advantage. There are many theories on the meaning of this phrase. Some say it's about confidence, others acting. If you don't feel confident, pretend you do until you gain the necessary skills or tools you need. Confidence is everything when playing the game of success. The only way to success is to believe it possible. Belief is a must. A mantra I apply during the day is, 'I have unwavering faith in me'. You must create unwavering faith, every moment of every day.

Amy Cuddy has taken this well-known phrase and put a twist on it: 'Don't fake it till you make it, fake it till you become it.' Let this quote land on you. What feelings does it inspire?

Being confident is not a prerequisite to achieving your outcomes. Knowing you want to become successful is your key to success. Remember, awareness is the key to change. Knowing your thoughts, your values, and your beliefs; knowing what your mountain top looks like, will build your confidence. Each moment builds your personal foundation, your personal belief, and your confidence in your vision.

'What is a mountain top?' It is your vision of where you believe your life can take you. It's your end goal, your pinnacle of achievement. You may call it your purpose. For me, purpose is what gets you up in the morning, your daily driving force, something you can no longer contain. My waking thoughts, my internal feelings, bubble over every morning with excitement and energy. Each day my focus is how to empower women to be their daily best. How to empower women to be their children's inspiration. Whereas my mountain top is the life dreams I hold for my family and myself. I long to live on a sandy beach, feeling peace and love within.

Can you see the difference? Can you differentiate between your purpose and your life mountain top?

I can feel anxiety and panic. Don't panic, my lovely friend. Allow time for the way ahead to reveal itself. Allow awareness to build and clarity to unfold. Give yourself the gift of asking yourself great questions and patiently waiting for your own answer. There is no going back from where you are at this moment. You have taken the lid off. It can, and will, be painful. I remember training for an Iron Man event and hearing this advice: 'It's not "Will it be painful?"; it's "When will it get painful?".'

Try as you might to put the lid back on the emotion – and you will try – it won't go back on; it can't go back on. It doesn't fit anymore. You are moving into a phase of self-discovery. Your authentic, true, self will become visible to you. This is the most exciting time of the learning process. The big reveal.

Kate's 'had enough moment'

Kate had been coming to indoor cycling classes with me for six months. She was new to fitness and excited to feel alive through exercise.

She approached me to personal train her in preparation for her first marathon. It is quite normal for me to train women in preparation for races, but not one who had registered for a marathon without any running experience. Kate could run for no longer than 90 seconds. One minute and 30 seconds was the longest time Kate could maintain running before she had to walk, totally out of breath. I love this. Let me just say again, with no experience or ability at that moment, Kate had entered a marathon. This makes me smile with love for the human spirit.

Kate had found a marathon plan but had no understanding of the jargon used or how to apply it to her life. In swoops Birdonabike.

From her first session my understanding of women became visible to Kate, and she felt her 'had enough' moment'. As she began to unpeel the layers of her thoughts, going deeper to her centre, Kate's senses became alive and emotions erupted. She was feeling and remembering life events that she had buried deep. All of those most inner thoughts came from asking simple, beautiful questions. She showed herself to herself. She hadn't known her reasons why she was drawn to run a marathon, merely the feeling of a great way to lose weight and get fit.

This hour session brought memories back that she had buried deep within her. Kate knew that this had opened a box that could never be shut. There could be no more deliberate memory loss, no more pretending that her relationships were straight out of *Cinderella* with birds singing, mice sewing and everyone living happily ever after.

She was running to be seen. She was running to feel she was enough. She was running to feel respected by all those around her, but more importantly to have love and respect for herself. Kate had had enough.

It was from this moment that I saw that training for events or races, looking good and feeling healthy, was never about the fitness. It was the feeling it gave women; the sense of purpose. For that moment she mattered. To have freedom of movement, to do something for herself; not be someone's mum or wife but to be free. To feel respected for an amazing achievement. To show that with vision, focus and action she was able to achieve her outcome, whatever that maybe.

The role of inspiring her family was born. She would be the breath of life.

Book trail

Forleo, M. (2008). *Make Every Man Want You: How to be so irresistible you'll barely keep from dating yourself!* New York: McGraw-Hill Contemporary. (Kindle edition available)

Ban Breathnach, S. (2007). *Romancing the Ordinary: A year of everyday indulgences.* New York: Simon & Schuster.

Ban Breathnach, S. (2012). *Peace and Plenty: Finding your path to financial security*. London: Corgi. (Kindle edition available)

7

The Body Never Lies

'When life gets you down, do you wanna know what you've gotta do? Just keep swimming!'

Dory, *Finding Nemo*

The body is your environment

Without health you have nothing. All the money and success you hold is like water in your hands.

To be successful you need a strong environment supporting and surrounding you. Your environment begins with your physiology: your body. This is your home. But we live in an age that does not support moving, an age of not- moving. We are far removed from our hunter-gatherer purpose.

Today's society encourages sedentary living. We drive cars, take lifts or escalators, and then we get home exhausted and slump on a comfy sofa watching TV. Our capacity for functional movement is deemed unnecessary. In our homes we have computers, laptops, and every up-to-date piece of equipment. The television is as large as we can fit in our rooms, with probably one in each of the bedrooms. The overstimulation of our senses is inhibiting our intelligence and diminishing our knowledge of the amazing world around us.

But wait, we exacerbate this numbing of our senses by having the TV on, volume blaring, while on the laptop, mobile phone beside us on the sofa, and we're taking photos to send to friends. Does that sound like you or your children? It drives me crazy. Have one on at a time!

Technology has transformed the way we move and communicate – not always for the better. A great example of this is when the children say they have spoken to their friends. They mean 'communicated with', not actually 'spoken to'. This always makes me have an internal chuckle. I have pulled back from correcting them; their perception is correct, but so is their mother's.

It is imperative that movement be a lifelong aspiration. It sounds obvious, but this is where I see the most resistance. Most women I have met have at some point in their lives expressed the wish to lose weight, get fit and tone up. But their goal is always for the immediate future, an instant result, not as an investment in their long-term future.

'Feeding luv'

Women share their thoughts and feelings about themselves with me daily. They beg for my support and help. They feel overwhelmed, exhausted. They have nothing left to give. They have exceptionally high aspirations for themselves and their families. They give to their family and friends first, leaving nothing for themselves. They have forgotten how to laugh, have fun, or even enjoy spending time with the people they love and adore the most. They question how it has come to this: despising the family they dreamed of having.

Their body image is rock bottom: they hate their wobbly tummies – their words, not mine. In fact, I have heard them describing their tummies as looking like cottage cheese or muffin tops. They loathe their flabby arms and call them – I hate this phrase – bingo wings. Last but by no means least, they hate their bums and thighs. I have had a request for a regime that would create a 'thigh gap'. These toxic thoughts about your body generate daily rituals that do not serve you well.

Weighing yourself daily: what's all that about? Does this daily practice reap rewards? In a word, *no!* You may have been truly focused on creating a body you will be happy with, or at least not hate; you've been dieting – well, starving yourself – for probably an age, decades, in fact; you're consumed with being slim or, even worse, skinny. You're exhausted.

You get on the scales – nothing lost. It's like groundhog day. This keeps happening. You must stop this.

Now is the time to build strength within you, through your thoughts and feelings. This will create a body flooded with love and energy. You will be a lighthouse, a beacon in the distance for people to follow.

Everybody will be drawn to you. You will have an abundance of energy, from your waking hour till dusk. There will be dips, of course, and fatigue, but you will have structures and knowledge to combat these trying times. The answer is always to give to yourself. I call it 'feeding luv'. You feed love to yourself first, then you have so much more to give others. Think of airlines going through their safety instructions: 'In an emergency place the oxygen mask over your own face before attending to children.' This always creates feelings that are challenging to process. It doesn't make sense to me on a mother level, but on a common sense level of course it makes sense.

Suzi's 'had enough' moment

Suzi was at breaking point. She was doing a wonderful job of masking her feelings. Really, she was overwhelmed, fatigued, full of self-loath, unable to enjoy relationships with her family, and she had forgotten how to laugh or have fun. Her range of moods had swung from periods of relative calmness to outbursts of anger. She couldn't understand why nobody could see through her Oscar-winning performance of coping. Why couldn't her husband see the state she was in? The fact is, he could. He even asked her if she was ok. Her reply? You guessed it: 'I'm fine'.

Her body was crying out for her to stop. Her weight was increasing, her skin pale-whitish, with dark sagging circles around the eyes. She didn't care what she looked like, or about her clothes or hair. Her presence had dwindled to nothing, no vibrations of energy around her. She made minimal eye contact, of course, as she didn't want people to see into her soul. Suzi came to me on her knees.

Firstly, we took an average day in her life and dissected it, bit by bit. She was very proud of the exercise she had incorporated into her life, from playing hockey in a local team to walking the dogs and running with her sister. We looked at her daily thoughts and what she felt like when she woke up. How did these feelings play out throughout the day? At no point in this initial stage did I analyze the extent of her exercise or her nutrition, I wanted to take away from Suzi's stressors, not add to them.

Exercise and controlled nutrition constitute stress on the body, guaranteeing failure. I repeat, exercise is stress on the body. You must get fit for fitness. Maybe this is a concept new to you, one that you resist. Suzi could not take any more physical activity, even if it was deemed healthy.

Suzi had a super-stressful job, one that she was unable to leave at the office. She brought the anxieties and stress back home with her and continued to work at home, even though she had three children and a husband. Literally nothing in Suzi's life was bringing her joy.

I asked Suzi these great questions:

- What are you aiming for?
- What do you want to feel like every day? Give me three feelings you want to experience on a daily basis.
- What do you think can help you move forward?
- Who is in your support network?

Her answers startled even her. She could not identify what she wanted and had no idea how she wanted to feel. What Suzi wanted was to be in control of her life again. More importantly, she wanted to feel again. She had become numb to life, numb to her emotions.

The strategies we discussed were simple but certainly not easy. We started one week at a time. First, she made a commitment to herself that no matter what time she got back from work, she was to leave the office behind and not do any more work at home.

You see, Suzi sometimes finished work at 16:00 but felt so guilty she continued to work on emails or administration on her return home. She never got back the extra hours she put in, so why the feelings of guilt?

Suzi found peace in her car, as she travelled between work locations. The car was Suzi's safe space in which to move from work to home life. This was a wonderful place to begin separating her work from home, giving

Suzi peace and time to heal from the day before going home to her loved family. I prescribed a ritual post-work of sitting in the car and allowing her thoughts to settle. Once settled, she would close her eyes and focus on her breath for one minute. I knew this practice would increase over time. Suzi had begun her journey of meditation: allowing peace and calm to enter her cellular structure, letting her busy mind settle and find peace. Suggesting to Suzi that she should meditate for 20 minutes a day would have set up resistance and felt as if I were adding to her workload. Starting with a minute was doable. It is a must to start from where you are, not where you think you should be. That minute was a must for debriefing from the day's work and allowing her mind to enter a peaceful state that would enhance her relationships within her family.

Each week we looked at Suzi's activities of daily living, tweaking behaviours rather than adding new ones. Wow – what a difference four weeks made! Life-changing!

If you feel resistance to adopting new behaviours, use your ABCs of awareness.

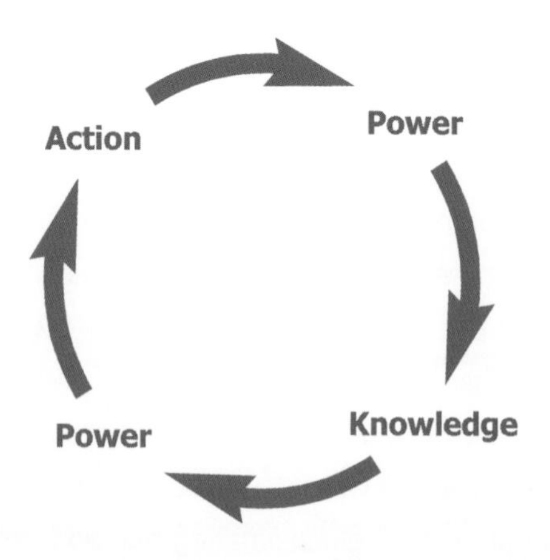

Using the Four-step Framework above, you can identify the stressors in your life and replicate the phases of Suzi's developing solution, aligning them to your issues.

But beware: although this is a useful prompt for building awareness, you must always look within first, and work on yourself before looking externally to others. It is always less challenging observing others than searching within yourself. This is where you will grow.

It is now time to ask yourself some great questions:

- What is my goal for this year for myself?
- What do I want to achieve this year?
- How do I want to feel each day?
- How do I want my body to look?
- How will that make me feel?
- Will I be able to recognize when I get to the result I have visualized?
- Do I want to drop a dress size or lose weight?
- Do I want to be weighed and how often?
- Do I want to take measurements of myself?
- Do I want to take 'before' and 'after' photos?
- Have I still got an old piece of clothing I want to get back into, such as smaller- sized jeans?
- How much time can I realistically commit to my outcome?
- Who is my support network?

ACTION

Take 5 minutes to write in your journal the answers to the great questions above.

If you have other questions related to your thoughts about your body, add them in too. How do I want my body to feel and look? Put this or any other question in your phone as a reminder, to come up at 2-hourly intervals. Throughout your day, allow yourself to answer the questions.

This technique will give you clarity of thought; it eliminates all the internal chatter and invests your vision of yourself with some reality. If you are realistic about what you want, the end result becomes more achievable. If you're a size 20 and your vision of yourself is to become a size 8 in a 12-week period, ask yourself if this is realistic. Guess what: *no*!

Don't do this to yourself. You know without me telling you that this is not a realistic outcome. I'm not being sizeist or negative. I'm being what you want me to be, and that is honest and trustworthy.

Use the 3 Bs:

1. Be honest
2. Be realistic
3. Be kind to yourself

I love your vision of reducing your dress size, and investing in your body and lifelong health, but you need to allow the time to achieve it, to be kind to yourself, and to be realistic.

I love being unrealistic, setting goals or entertaining dreams that I think are impossible, yet believing in them anyway. But this would be taking the concept out of context. Be kind to yourself, and be realistic about your body.

Investing time in your self-vision is the foundation for progress. Keeping the vision alive will require you to write down your daily thoughts and feelings. Believe me, the mind is amazing at trickery. It will forget the feelings you had about your body unless you capture them.

I say it again, write them down and put a date to your writing. When you read them back, you won't believe you ever felt like that about yourself and the world you live in. You will doubt the written evidence, 'Is that how I truly felt?'

Book trail

Banks, S. (2012). *Missing Link: Reflections on Philosophy and Spirit.*

Franklin, E. (2003). *Pelvic Power: Mind/Body exercises for strength, flexibility posture and balance for men and women.* New York: Princeton Book Company.

Guiliano, M. (2006). French Women Don't Get Fat: The secret of eating for pleasure. London: Vintage. (Kindle edition available)

8

Build Your Foundations Deep

'It doesn't matter where you start.
Your only limit is your soul.'
Chef Gusteau, *Ratatouille*

Posture

Before you think of transforming your body with amazing nourishing foods, or weekly exercise, think posture, do posture, be a peacock.

I remember, years ago, researching alternative methods to weight loss and the relation of happiness to weight loss. I came across Paul McKenna's book, *I Can Make You Happy*. I loved his first technique – part of his instant pick-me-ups. He called it the 'Happy Posture'. What a wonderful thought: that simply standing – and being – more present in your body could begin the process of happiness.

Posture is the foundation of your movement. Aligning your body correctly, and maintain that alignment, creates positive body language. It's like the peacock displaying his feathers, saying 'look at me'.

If your eyes are the gateway to your soul, your posture is the title of your story. I have been observing people for 20 years. Watching with awe their individual ability to create movement through the placement of their feet on the ground. I can tell what a person's posture will look like simply by the way they land their foot. This vital insight shows me the person within, their thoughts, their feelings, their strengths and the challenges in their daily life.

ACTION

Take two minutes to reflect and write your answers in your journal.

- How does my foot land on the ground?
- How does my foot roll and push off the ground?
- What happens to the rest of my body when my foot strikes the ground?
- How does my body feel when my foot strikes?
- Have I got any pain during foot placement?

This will give you a great base to start looking at your body's foundation and an insight into your posture.

Your body reflects your thoughts. The mind and body are connected. Your physical body vibrates with energy at a cellular level. How you align your body from the foot strike has an impact on the flow of energy through your body.. It's a simple alignment from the top of your head to the base of your foot. You align your own energy pathways.

Let's go a bit 'woowoo' with ancient traditions. I used to fear 'woowoo'; now I'm finding new knowledge and applications of the ancient art of 'woowoo'! To reach self-mastery we must align our physical, emotional and spiritual energies. It is vital to our aim of being extraordinary, of being our daily best.

Chakras and meridians are pathways of energy that run through the body to create inner balance, and they are connected to the vital organs around the body. Chakra is a Sanskrit (the primary liturgical language of Hinduism) word for 'wheel'. There are seven major energy centres throughout the body. They are aligned along the spinal column and connected to our physical, emotional, spiritual and mental wellbeing.

Meridians are invisible channels of energy, each with a beginning and an end. Meridians and acupoints date from ancient 2658 BCE, in China. They flow into one another, each conducting their own energy known, as 'qi' pronounced 'chi'. I became familiar with this term from an Aikido Master I trained. We often debated cellular connectivity and proprioception (the body's perception of its position in the space around it). I have him to thank for returning me to the art of centering.

The imbalance of chakra and meridian alignment creates 'dis-ease'. This makes wonderful sense to me. It always makes me smile: despite all our research and knowledge, the ancient traditions display an instinctive awareness of how their bodies work compared with our ignorance today. Ignorance definitely is never bliss.

Your posture is the key to your whole being. Posture supports our emotions and our physiology, and it nourishes our spirit.

The ancient martial arts, yoga, Pilates, and modern techniques, such as Bowen Technique, Alexander Technique, etc., develop balance and strength. I have been practising Pilates for the past 16 years and have the privilege of teaching both classic and modern styles of Pilates. I am truly passionate about supporting people to move with purpose and ease.

Pilates was created by Joseph Pilates in the early 20th century. He was a sickly child and he created a method to aid his own personal health, combining kung fu, yoga, gymnastics, and bodybuilding. He developed these further to create 'Contrology', a method of mind controlling muscle. It focuses on core postural strength and precision of movement. Pilates has grown into one of the most popular fitness techniques of the 21st century. There are many different schools of Pilates, each with its own understanding of the original works.

Teaching mixed ability groups – age is not a factor or a hindrance – to develop their own personal Pilates practice is rewarding. I have been teaching one of my classes for nine years and 80% of its members have been with me from the beginning. They are the most proficient and effective in the way they move. Their average age is 68, so they are clearly fulfilling my dreams of lifelong mobility and health.

I believe in creating a foundation for your health to build on. Pilates will give you this strong foundation.

With all new clients, regardless of their goals, postural strength, awareness and precision of movement. Breathing techniques are invaluable for ADLs. Pilates has supported people to adapt their running techniques and to build life skills for the reducing injuries that come to challenge us daily.

Postural tips

Here is a brief guide to achieving a strong standing posture

- Do not move into any posture that causes you pain.
- Breathe deep and wide into your ribcage.
- Be conscious of your body and your movement.
- Stand with your feet hip-distance apart.
- Feel your feet connect to the earth, weight placed equally on the big toe, little toe, and heel.
- Shift your weight forward and backward, and then centre your weight through your feet.
- Bend your knees slightly, then slightly lengthen the legs, being mindful not to push the knees too open to the point where you feel pressure on the backs of the knees.
- Hips are set directly in line with the ankle, balanced above the feet.
- Pull up on your pelvic floor.
- Engage your abdominals, but do not brace them.
- Your ribcage is centred over your hips and connected to them, creating abdominal strength.
- Do not flare the ribcage; this will affect your lower back.
- Your shoulder blades are engaged and down, but not forced; you should feel that the bottom tips of the shoulder blades are activated.
- Lengthen your neck, drawing the ears away from the shoulders.

This posture is a working base. It is challenging to maintain, and the skill of keeping this form while moving is no less challenging. But it feels strong. It feels balanced. It gives a sense of power.

Social psychologist Amy Cuddy's TED talk discussed how body language could shape who we are. She introduced the Power Pose, the result of a wonderful piece of research she conducted. The Power Pose is a standing posture that, when maintained for two minutes, has a demonstrable effect on hormone levels. It changes your body chemistry, and has an impact on confidence and possible success.

The Power Pose is based on the body language of winning athletes as they cross the finishing line. Just picture that open 'look at what I have done' pose. The talk suggests adopting this open 'X'-shaped pose two minutes before an important meeting or interview to build confidence and an air of authority. What this research revealed was that we could change people's perception of us just by our body language.

I applied this technique to pre-race rituals for clients and for myself. My results were outstanding. I now suggest to clients that they adopt this position before their personal training sessions and then they are at their peak. Tony Robbins calls this your 'peak state'.

Being able to shift state is a skill, but it can be actioned in a moment. This sounds so simple, but it is super-challenging when you're absolutely at rock bottom.

The energy postural alignment creates is explosive. It's such a powerful skill to use and develop. Music is also a wonderful state changer. It can take postural alignment to the next level of purposeful movement. This powerful, progressive, body language must be practised and incorporated into your ADLs.

ACTION

In a peaceful space, take two minutes to ask yourself these questions:

- Why do I weigh myself?
- How do I feel before and after weighing?
- How regularly do I weigh myself?

Write your findings in your journal.

Rebecca's 'had enough' moment

What a warm, giving, caring, adorable personality I welcomed into my Pilates class! But soon I came to understand Rebecca's battle with her self-image and weight – and it was a battle. Daily she destroyed her soul with her internal chatter. She expressed to me her utter disdain for herself. She felt large, wobbly, unattractive and too visible to the world.

Rebecca's personal training with me began with such excitement. Her determination was off the scale. We trained together twice weekly, with Rebecca going to her gym in the interim. But the amazing impetus she had put behind her vision quickly evaporated. She stopped training as her busy family commitments did not allow her to give an hour to herself.

At her second attempt at personal training the results started to show. She lost weight weekly, and there were visible changes to her body and her energy. Her support network resisted these changes out of misguided affection, but this undermined her training momentum. A tempting glass of wine on her return from work, fast food on days out with kids, and takeaways soon meant that the weight loss was no more. A wonderful husband who 'loved her just the way she was' didn't help either. Her efforts were just not rewarding her enough and soon she stopped training again.

On returning to personal training for a third time, she realised the extent of her her weight obsession. She weighed herself every day. It was like a self-abuse ritual. She weighed herself every day even when she had not implemented any change behaviour. Albert Einstein said, 'Insanity is doing the same thing over and over again and expecting different results.'

On top of our twice-weekly session, I suggested a catch-up, to demonstrate to her the potential strength of her willpower, as this was something she was blind to. As she struggled with the mini battles within her social world, we designed strategies together to maximize her chances of success.

The jeans strategy worked beautifully. Rebecca had a pair of jeans that she was desperate to get back into. They were two sizes smaller than her present size. She brought them out, and asked her family to come together for a family meeting. She explained her vision to them all, asking for their support and guidance. The jeans were to go into every room that she went into. They lay on the back of her kitchen chairs, perfect as a physical reminder of her dream. This was a wonderfully concrete reminder for both Rebecca and her supportive family.

ACTION

Take 2 minutes to think of a piece of clothing you would love to slide back into – not squeeze, slide.

(You could use a photo, but actually having a piece of clothing in your hand, something tactile, will bring your goal to life.)

It has to be something that you love, truly would do anything to fit back into. It's usually a pair of jeans. Who doesn't want to fit back into their pre-baby jeans? Find the piece of clothing that you loved before babies, or that you felt like a million dollars in that you loved wearing, or that you always got the most amazing compliments in.

Write your thoughts in your journal and date them.

Book trail

Pilates, J.H. and Miller, W.J. (2014). *Return to Life through Contrology*. Eastford, CT: Martino Fine Books.

9

Daily Rituals

'Venture outside of your comfort zone.
The rewards are worth it.'

Rapunzel, *Tangled*

This chapter is super-powerful. It will create a foundation for your life to help you to grow into your dreams.

GROW into the genius of your body.
GROW into the extraordinary life that is there for you to invest in.
GROW into a lifetime love affair with you.

ACTION

Take 2 minutes to let these words land on you. Acknowledge them, and become aware of the feelings that come from within

- What do you feel?
- How do you feel it in your body?
- Where in the body?

Write your thoughts in your journal and date them.

Finding your purpose

My gift to you is to this: 'Listen to your Body. It is genius.'

Know that you may feel totally uncomfortable, but know that greatness will come from feeling this way; your body is feeding back to you.

Daily rituals are part of the process of mastering personal wisdom. They create discipline on a consistent daily basis. This in turn will shift you into the success that you have only seen in your dreams. Daily rituals are conscious daily actions implemented to create habits that pave your way to success.

Jim Rohn has said, 'Motivation is what gets you started. Habit is what keeps you going.'

Habits are your memorized state of being. Habits are your body automatically doing something that the mind set in motion years ago. Habits are part of your personality. They are the way you think, act and choose to behave. Habits are your behaviours.

Dr Dispenza proclaims, 'The biggest habit to break is being yourself.'

You may be thinking to yourself 'What do you mean by rituals?' Let me explain. Daily rituals are consistent, conscious, chosen behaviours used every day to create power within you. Imagine building the deepest, strongest, widest foundations to base your vision on. These foundations will support whatever life throws at them. These foundations will withstand the toughest of weathers and the most challenging of times. Daily rituals will be the pathway to your purpose – the purpose that you think about most in the day. The purpose that you wake up with, vibrating with excitement in every cell.

I know what you're going to say next: 'What if I don't have a purpose?'

'What if I have no idea what my purpose is?'

ACTION

Please use your journal. Writing gets your thoughts right into the nervous system till they become part of you.

I will support you with this black hole of a question.

'If you did know your purpose, what would your answer be?'

Listen to your body. Listen to the first words that come to you. Write them down. *Now.* Take no longer than 5 minutes.

Enjoy this. Smile as you are writing. This may not come easily to you. The writer in you, the chronicler of your life, maybe lying dormant within.

DO NOT freeze.
DO NOT fear.
DO NOT judge yourself.

Listen to your body, and return to the breath. Just breathe

You are giving yourself one of the greatest gifts. You are building your extraordinary life. You are building the pathway to what you truly want to give to life.

Dr Wayne Dyer takes away the pain of finding your purpose in his story documentary *The Shift*. We do not have to have a given purpose. Every human's divine purpose is to contribute, to serve others.

Your purpose is to contribute

I love this. It takes my breath away. It's an inner valve releasing personal pressure. It makes sense to me.

YES, we are unique.
YES, we have individual gifts.
YES, we all have something to offer the world.

But the pressure we and the world of personal development place on us creates pain within, creates resistance and choice. It's as if the world is saying, 'You can choose what you want your gift to be, but choose wisely as this might not be the unique gift given to you and you will have wasted all that time and effort investing in a gift that was never yours.'

Having to choose will always lead to inaction. Give a human too much choice and they will be paralyzed.

Listen to your body and the feelings that arise when you take away the pressure of searching for your purpose, and you replace the search with the feeling of knowing. Knowing that your purpose is to contribute creates inner harmony.

YOU already know how it feels to contribute.
YOU already know the physical changes that occur when you support people.
YOU already know that this is your purpose, to contribute.

Daily rituals will provide you with the comfort of inner strength, knowledge of yourself, and a place to return to when things become too much to bear. Oh, and they will. Please know this, I will always be honest with you.

So what rituals occupy your day?

ACTION

Find a quiet peaceful time in your day. Take no longer than 5 minutes to write your daily routine down in your journal, looking at three non-consecutive days. Are there any similarities between them? Remember, knowledge is power.

These are exciting times: you have heightened your awareness of your daily routine. Awareness is the key to change. To become aware of yourself will give you clarity. Clarity is part of the process to becoming able to perform at the highest level and then maintaining that level of performance.

I continually study great leaders, the super-successful, and model the most extraordinary businesses in the universe. I study their strategies, the systems they have implemented, and the tools they use to measure results/outcomes. From the very beginning, all the individuals have a clear vision of the outcomes want, and how they want to feel and behave towards themselves and others. They have a plan or model, which has been set out from the beginning, but it constantly adapts to changing circumstances to make sure their vision is achievable. They all carry out daily rituals, from the time they get up in the morning to when they go to bed, via the sequence of behaviours they implement before setting off to work.

I am going to share with you my daily rituals.

Rituals maketh the man

Bird's Morning Rituals

1. Rise for the magic hour of 05:00–06:00.
2. Drink 500 ml clean quality water.
3. Meditate with Chicken 20–30 minutes. (Chicken is my cat. I adore her.)
4. 10 minutes of rebounding/lymphasizing, with daily affirmations said aloud. Laugh/smile.
5. Write down what is important to me today and who to contact.
6. Fasting exercise as part of my training plan (unless I am exercising for over 90 minutes), or fasting walk for a minimum of 20 minutes.
7. Open body up: 10/10/10 (minutes on each)
8. Stimulating body brushing.
9. Beautiful breakfast. Putting goodness inside, fuelling the body. This is my favourite meal of the day. I love how it makes me feel and I get very, very excited.

Bird's Evening Rituals

10. Go to bed 3 hours after eating. You must go to bed hungry.
11. Daily reflection (and conscious breathing) for 2 minutes; writing up my gratitude diary and preparing for tomorrow.

I've shown you my day, but I'm not saying, 'Wow, look at me, aren't I great?' I've done it to illustrate my dedication and commitment to my vision, my dreams, and the discipline and love I invest in my purpose and myself. It is an absolute must that I devote daily time to dream-making.

Think of yourself as an artist, creating a new picture depicting your vision. You are creating a 4D approach to your life:

1. Your dream: this is visual stimulus
2. Your devotion: this is the emotion stimulus
3. Your determination: this is the momentum stimulus
4. Your discipline: this is the power stimulus

Your dreams are a vital energy force for your life. Without dreams there are no life adventures for you. Without the purpose of pursuing adventures, you are motionless. You do not move, forward, backward, or in any direction. Without movement, without motion there is no energy. Without energy – the life force – what is there?

Energy = Living

It is your duty to be fit, lean and healthy. It is your duty to unite mind, body and spirit. It is your duty to achieve inner health and a wealth of energy.

Plutarch, the Greek historian and philosopher, wrote 'What we achieve inwardly will change outer reality.'

ACTION

This exercise takes 5 minutes. It's all about you. Take a deep breath in and ask yourself:

- What is my dream?
- What is my life vision?
- What is my purpose?

Breathe. Let the words land on you.

Now write down your answers and date them. This may feel 'sticky' but it's awesome. This is super-simple but not easy. You may feel frustration, but let the words breathe through you.

If you have ever practised yoga or stretched your body in, flexibility classes, You will know it can be 'sticky' in some places in your body. You know your body is able to move and stretch, but it won't do it without practice. You have to breathe to get the muscles to release.

If you are not able to let go of your frustration, when you are breathing, use words to help you. Words used as a way of supporting the body are called mantras. A mantra is a wonderful tool. When breathing in say in your mind 'open'; when breathing out say in your mind 'release'.

Do this for no more than 10 minutes.

Dedication and determination are powerful qualities required to create momentum. Without these elements your dream will have 'no legs'. It will remain a dream, as so many do.

Your discipline comes from your thoughts and consistent daily behaviour. Chosen daily rituals that you have total faith in will lead you to your dream.

Discipline entails implementing the actions even though it may be painful, even though it goes against everything your internal chatter is persuading you to do. Discipline is getting up early on a cold, wet morning because you have total belief in your dream.

Discipline keeps the faith, when potentially everyone around you says 'no'.

I'm going to share with you my 11 daily rituals. They are super-simple, but be under no illusion: it may take some time for you to absorb them into your everyday routine.

Daily Ritual 1: the 5 o'clock club

Wake up at 05:00. (I can feel the resistance already!)

Set your alarm. When you hear it, you will feel exhausted. Don't worry, this is to be expected. You won't want to get up. Don't worry, this is also to be expected. Be warned, if you 'snooze' when the alarm goes off for the second time you will slightly feel more tired; if you hit another 'snooze' failure is just around the corner. Say goodbye to your morning preparation.

I confess, I sometimes snooze; this is fatal. The mind plays tricks; it coerces you and fools you into thinking that staying in bed and resting are better for you than getting up. Don't allow the resistance in your mind to win: *get up!*

Congratulate yourself for beginning the day with your greatest gift to yourself: the 'magic hour'. Tony Robbins calls this the 'power hour'. Call it what you will, for me, this is where the magic happens, where my unconscious mind is allowed to breathe, think and imprint its thoughts into my being, where exercise feeds my soul.

Now, once you are up, maybe not yet fully awake, you will see jobs around the house that might distract you. Your household's potential to distract you cannot be overestimated. It talks to you, telling you you are being selfish in going out to exercise while there is so much to be done in the house. Starting now will put you ahead in your day. No!

I hope you can hear me supporting you not to listen to your internal chatter. Nothing good will come from this moment of distraction. You have been truly amazing in getting up at this hour of the morning, so don't let anything get in the way of feeding your soul with movement.

Another challenge you may find, are the loved ones around you: partners, children, family members, friends, and colleagues. They love you. They, of course, have their values and beliefs, which they will share with you. Observe their reactions to the change in your behaviours. They will react; they are only human. Respect their humanity and remember that what they say to you always comes with the best of intentions.

My advice is always to set goals that you can achieve. This daily ritual is super-challenging. It may take some time to be able to get up that early. You will fail. This is what athletes call training to failure. You are taking your body beyond its current capabilities, but don't worry. Your body will adapt. You will grow. You will succeed.

I have recently had shoulder surgery, following a bike accident last year. Two days after the operation, I set my alarm for 0500. It was a must for me to re-introduce it into my ADLs. Even if I couldn't exercise it was important that my morning routine return to its peak state. I only didn't get up if the pain was too great or if I had not slept enough the previous night. I set the alarm and got up. As my body recovered, I was soon back in the daily ritual of 05:00 'The Magic Hour'.

Not only are you investing in your health, but you're also gaining hours in the day. Remember, all the greatest leaders and achievers have the same 24 hours as us mere mortals; it's just that they find more productive hours in their day. Getting up at 05:00 gives you a two-hour head start on the day; that equates to an extra 728 hours in a year. Look at what you could achieve with those extra hours.

Ask yourself this great question: how much more could I achieve if I had another 2 hours in the day? Hey, ask an amazing question, get a great answer.

The magic hour

The hours between 0:500 and 06:00 or 06:00 and 07:00 hold energy like no other time of day. The energy is visible: it distorts the vibrations from the earth; you can feel it at a cellular level within you and hear the sounds echo throughout the sky.

At this hour, the universe is at peace. The energy and its vibrations are balanced. I visualize a porthole of light entering my centre. I feel plugged into the universe; this is the time for my womanly power to flourish: all is well with the world and you bestow peace on the community around you.

Most people are sleeping and miss the world unveiling itself to the day. Amazing things happen to you at this hour.

You smile and greet people with a 'hello! They smile and greet you back. This simple exchange of small gestures creates such vibrations of energy within us. The more I become aware of the world, I not only look, but also I see. I not only listen, but I also hear. I not only touch, but I also feel.

I see myself.
I hear myself
I matter to me.
I will make a difference today.

ACTION

Set your alarm for 05:00. Acknowledge your personal resistance to this and potentially that of your loved ones. You may start talking yourself out of this practice the night before! When you resist change or transformation, you become the greatest storyteller in the world. I have one word to say to you: *don't*! Get into this daily habit of setting your alarm for 05:00.

Everything I teach and support always starts at your beginning, where you are today.

It's like Julie Andrews sings in *The Sound of Music*: 'Let's start at the very beginning; it's a very good place to start.' Come on!

But please listen to your body and be realistic. If you are starting from a normal habit of getting up after 09:00 in the morning, please be kind to yourself. Adopt this new ritual gradually so you can achieve it. It does not make sense to go straight to 05:00. Start with 08:00. Each week make it one hour earlier. Before you know it, you will have introduced this amazing ritual without creating immediate resistance to adaptation. If you reduce your resistance, you reduce the risk of failing to create new habits.

OK, now you're up, what do you do?

And so it begins, my friends

Daily Ritual 2: Drink beautiful quality water

Hydrate: give your body a morning boost to its energy by drinking a glass of water – it's a super-simple Daily Ritual. If it's so simple, then why is it the most ignored basic need for the body to survive? This is a hugely important part of my assessment of health and energy levels in the body: 90% of the thousands of people I have had the honour to teach either drink none or not enough water during their day. I know, it's unbelievable, but easily done.

Remember, we are busy being busy being busy.

Claire's 'had enough' moment

Claire is a wonderful lady, a young mum of one, slender, and loves to run by herself. She runs alone to keep fit and keep her figure. She has a great career, but now works it around the family. She has been attending Pilates classes for about two months, feeling the need to build length and strength into her body. At the end of class Claire chats to me about her running, her love for the great outdoors, and how it makes her feel. It gives her time to think and breathe. It's definitely not about competing or challenging her body.

During the last two or three runs she has felt sluggish. She didn't enjoy the runs; in fact, she hated them. She was so disappointed with herself. You see, the end result is never the guarantor to happiness. It's the feelings along the way that count. You will see this pattern appearing time and time again, throughout each of these personal stories.

Claire and I informally discussed her daily routines, nutrition, sleep, stress. None of them seemed to hold the key to her training fatigue. We even got to the stage of her writing out a food diary, but there was no need. Her nutrition was spot-on. The culprit? Water – or lack of it.

Claire hates water. How can anyone hate water?

I get it, though. We know it's a necessity of life, but some people find it boring and tasteless, and some even put conditions on it: it must be cold or room temperature, flavoured, fizzy or still, and the list goes on.

Claire realized that she probably only drank 300ml of water during the day. She drank lots of tea and coffee, some fruit juice and no alcohol.

Simply starting to drink water changed her training into a magic hour, giving massive boost to her energy levels. Running has become blissful, connecting back to herself, her surroundings and her breath. Something so simple made a huge impact on her life!

The European Food Safety Authority (EFSA) recommends an intake of 2.5 litres of water for men and 2.0 litres of water for women per day. (The NHS expresses this as 8 x 200 ml glasses for women and 10 glasses for men.

This changes when you exercise: keeping hydrated before and after exercise Can require added supplements specific to your outcome/goals. This depends on the duration of the exercise. You must be hydrated before exercising. It is a matter of personal physiology, but you should take a few sips every 20 minutes.

ACTION

Take one large glass (250ml minimum) of water (filtered or tap) and drink.

To take this further, add fresh lemon.

To take this further still, add fresh lemon to a 250ml glass of water and leave overnight, ready to kick-start your body in the morning.

This idea of leaving the lemon in overnight first came about when I worked with Sophia Villiers, women's expert nutritionist. We discussed at length how to make the most of this simple practice.

There is conflicting research to show that the effect of lemon juice on the teeth can impair the enamel and create sensitivity. If your teeth begin to feel sensitive when drinking lemon water, use a straw to bypass the problem. This will make you smile in the morning, as you revert to your inner child.

It is vital that you understand your thoughts and feelings about this simple ritual:

- What are you thinking about when you drink?
- Are you thinking or are you just doing?
- What do you believe drinking is doing to your body?

Would knowing the impact water makes on your energy levels change the way you think about water?

It is the most wonderful source of energy, and without it we could not exist.

I am keeping the practice of hydration simple, to provoke the least resistance. But the process of drinking water can become complex when you analyse the quality and cleanliness of water.

I have been on the hunt for many a year for the most efficient water system for the home and for travelling. Please tell me that you are asking yourself 'What's wrong with tap water?' I'm with you on that one, but all is not what it seems. In the UK our tap water is not of the purest of quality, and we need to take personal responsibility for providing quality water for our families. What is in the water can have a profound effect on our energy production. The toxins and hormones found in tap water can block the energy efficiency of the cells.

I cannot urge you enough to drink more glorious water. It is a readily available energy source, waiting for you to pour it into your daily life.

Steps in progressing this ritual

It's simple: first, **Drink more water** – can you hear me inspiring you with love?

Then, when you have begun to enjoy drinking water and increased your daily intake, ask yourself, 'How can I provide my family with the highest quality water?'

There are many options available, from simple water filter jugs to ionizers installed in your home – systems that alter the ions in the water to enable your body to be more efficient in producing energy. There are also drops that alter the pH (acidity) of the water.

In our home we use a wonderful water system: Eva Advanced Water Filtration System (7 litre size). It removes all the potentially noxious elements in our tap water, chlorine, bacteria and heavy metals to name a few. After eliminating these harmful substances, it remineralizes through the volcanic rock layer. It looks magnificent.

Daily Ritual 3: Connect to your breath

How do you feel about spending time with yourself? Just sitting. Just breathing. Some might call this meditation, but I want to keep this simple.

Whenever I talk about meditation it summons up feelings that are hard to dispel. I hear lots of responses to the challenges of meditation.

1. 'I don't have time to just sit there and do nothing.'
2. 'I hate sitting still.'
3. 'My mind doesn't stop thinking.'
4. 'It's boring.'
5. 'I have children; they don't give me any space.'

'Meditation is difficult; it's supposed to be.' These are not my words, but the words of Ram Das, the world-renowned spiritual leader. And I would definitely agree with him.

I have found the practice of meditation daunting, but I have always been drawn to it through my love of yoga. I adore yoga. I have for the past two years had weekly one-to-one yoga sessions. I believe in purposeful conscious movement. I'm also a Pilates teacher, so breathing is the essence of my movement. Within the breath I connect to my physiology, I become aware of my physical body, its range, and its abilities.

I have deliberately not used the term 'limitations'. I do not wish to draw my attention to my limitations, only to how much my body can achieve.

I developed a pathway to meditation through bite-size chunks: I started with one minute of meditation. I built on this very quickly. I found myself longing to spend more time in that state. I didn't label it meditation, but breathing, self-connection, me-time instead.

You will see that this is a pattern of mine. I identify my personal clarity and listen to it. I research how to be more extraordinary and then listen to my feelings: how does it make me feel? If I feel resistance, I acknowledge it and create a process that will give me the desired result. Always.

I originally felt overwhelmed with 'making time' to meditate. I therefore started with small, very small, allocations of time and built on my personal foundation.

The benefits of connecting to yourself to your source are endless, especially in this age of distraction, busyness and resistance. If anything, connection with our being, our surroundings, our love, is needed more than ever. With meditation, your physiology undergoes cellular change. Your energy levels increase.

Meditation deactivates your 'fight or flight' response, enabling you to switch into your 'rest and digest' mode. These are two opposing nervous responses within your body.

'Fight or flight' is a primal stress response. It would be vital for survival if a sabre-toothed tiger were chasing you, but those days are gone. In this mode our nervous system releases hormones such as adrenaline and cortisol, which break the body down over time. The demands on our energy are immense, which leaves you feeling fatigued, perhaps with that 'crashed and burned' feeling. Inevitably, the immune system is also depleted.

The 'rest and digest' mode activates healing and regeneration. Low levels of adrenaline and cortisol create a sense of peace and balance within. This mode activates the more tranquil functions of the body. It is vital to spend more time in 'rest and digest' mode than 'fight or flight' mode.

Here are 20 benefits of meditation, physiological, emotional and spiritual.

1. Reduces anxiety
2. Increases exercise tolerance
3. Improves concentration and attention
4. Reduces stress
5. Lowers cholesterol
6. Saves energy
7. Cures headaches and migraines
8. Lowers the risk of cardiovascular disease
9. Slows the ageing process
10. Helps with weight loss
11. Helps to build sexual energy and desire
12. Increases emotional stability
13. Builds self-confidence
14. Speeds falling asleep, so cures insomnia
15. Changes attitude towards life
16. Increases acceptance of self
17. Brings body, mind and spirit into harmony
18. Develops intuition
19. Increases productivity
20. Increases creativity

ACTION

Immediately after getting up at 05:00, find a place to sit, either in your bed or on a particular chair. Make this a place where you consciously breathe. Sit upright, in a relaxed, open body position, with your hands resting gently in your lap, the palms facing down or up to the universe. If you feel you need all the energy you can get, keep your palms down. If you feel the environment needs it, keep your palms up.

Set an alarm for 2 minutes. If you feel this is far too long, start with 1 minute. Trust me, it will go so fast that you will soon progress your practice to 2 minutes.

During this session, do one thing only:

BREATHE

If thoughts come into your mind – to-do lists, worries, anxieties, stresses – don't worry:

BREATHE

This is not the time to ask yourself great meaningful questions like, what is my purpose in life? No...

JUST BREATHE

You will grow to love these 2 minutes. Remember, breathing is moving.

Once you have begun this meditation, the simplicity of it will give you such a wonderful feeling, you will spontaneously increase the time.

Each day, increase the time by a minute. Before you know it, you will have created a daily routine of ten minutes.

I have now developed my session into a minimum of 20 minutes. My cat Chicken also has discovered the benefits of meditation. When she sees me sitting upright and putting a scarf over my lap, that's her cue 'assume the position' and she leaps onto my lap and takes up her coma mode.(There is so much written about animals and meditation.)

I love being wrong; truly, it makes me smile. Therefore, when I think I can't or won't do a task, I find a way through. This is true of meditation. I kept telling myself for years that I couldn't sit still, that I couldn't still my creative active mind, let alone my busy body. I was wrong. Yay! I devised strategies that enabled me to find a way through.

Now it is unthinkable to not schedule this practice into my day. Meditation is an absolute must for action. It is like oxygen to me. I couldn't be without it.

Daily Ritual 4: Rebounding/lymphasizing/bouncing

This has to be my favourite 10 minutes of the day. You are going to love this: bouncing on a mini indoor trampoline! I mean, who doesn't love to bounce?

I was introduced to the practice of bouncing while I was in Brighton in August 2012, on a Tony Robbins 9-day course on becoming a master of personal wealth and health – yes, nine days. One of the maddest nine days of my life, but I gained some extraordinary lifelong friends from this experience.

We detoxed for the first five super-long days, indoors with no windows in the middle of summer. It was shorts weather outside, but jumpers and jeans, hats and gloves weather indoors. I was supposed to be training for a marathon – well, that went out of the window.

If you've ever been to a Tony Robbins experience, you'll know that it is extraordinary: the energy in the room, the hopes and fears, the anticipation and excitement. This level of energy is sustained by having mini trampolines around outside the massive function rooms. When you feel yourself dropping in focus or energy, you are prompted to use them. And they work.

On leaving the course I bought my own mini trampoline, not an expensive one, and began my daily ritual of bouncing. I have fallen in love with it.

I'm fit, with great health, I'm motivated and committed, but when I first started, five minutes was exhausting. My calf muscles ached – it was sheer pain at times. I got slightly breathless. Who would have believed that I had done an Ironman challenge if they'd seen what I was like after all of 5 minutes on the mini trampoline? When I got off the trampoline I felt like Bambi struggling to take his first steps. But as the momentum I put into this daily practice grew, so did my endurance.

Now I do 10 minutes, regardless of what may follow in my day; whether I'm personal training with clients, or training myself for an event, I bounce. There used to be some mornings when I really couldn't think of anything worse. It all seemed like too much effort. Whenever I sense my mind and body feeling agitated, I always stop, take a breath in and out, and then move forward into my scheduled ritual. Be committed to your schedule.

Within seconds of starting bouncing the boost to my energy is remarkable. Now it's your turn.

ACTION

Set your alarm. I always use the timer on my mobile. Set it for 5 minutes when you're starting the practice, increasing each day until you have built up to 10 minutes.

Now bounce: if you want to do star jumps or chuck in some shapes, it's your choice.

Have fun with this practice. Laugh, sing, enjoy.

Do not have any distractions. Tell your family not to disturb you, unless the house is on fire..

I was surprised to see how much information there is on rebounding. Even NASA has published scientific studies comparing the impact on the body from bouncing and running to G-forces.

I initially started this practice in pursuit of the health benefits of lymphasizing. Lymphasizing relates to the activity of the lymph system. The lymph system transports immune cells round the body and plays a major part in supporting a healthy immune system. Lymphasizing specifically stimulates the flow of lymph fluid through the system. The changes in gravity while you are bouncing produce a greater flow, leading to an increase in the waste and toxins flushed from the body.

Rebounding is often suggested as a detoxifying and immunity-boosting activity.

'Rebounding allows the muscles to go through the full range of motion at equal force. It helps people learn to shift their weight properly and to be aware of body positions and balance,' says James White, Ph.D., Director of Research and Rehabilitation in the Physical Education Department, University of California at San Diego. By jumping up and down you are actually cleansing your cells and detoxifying your system. By having clean cells without the toxic build up, your energy levels increase dramatically, allowing all the cells in your body to function efficiently.

I have suggested you do a 10-minute session, but please feel free to increase your sessions to up to an hour. Be aware that increasing bouncing time transforms this practice from daily lymphasizing into a fitness activity. When you're increasing your fitness endurance it's wise go for no more than a 10% increase in effort every week. Please be kind to your body.

I'm always keen to put my daily 24 hours to the most effective use. Therefore, while you are bouncing, say out loud to the universe through affirmations or mantras that you are amazing. Saying it out loud builds cellular belief and develops your thoughts and your personal faith in your life's journey.

I use affirmations and mantras when I bounce. I affirm that my purpose is to support people. How best I can support and teach them. In this way I connect with my desired core feelings. An affirmation is a declaration that something is true.

Gabrielle Bernstein, in *May Cause Miracles,* takes you through a process using different affirmations every day to declare your truth to the universe. If you are spiritual, this practice will be familiar to you. If this is all new to you, you're probably thinking this is all a bit 'woowoo'.

Some of these practices will take you way out of your comfort zone and make you feel very uncomfortable. This is where it gets exciting. Moving out of your comfort zone can be hugely challenging, but this is how you will stretch yourself and grow. Always listen to yourself: if you feel painful resistance, acknowledge it and devise a strategy to get round it. Start with just rebounding first, build the practice up in time, then – and only then – drop in an uplifting mantra with personal meaning.

Within 10 seconds of starting to bounce, I'm smiling and energy vibrates through my body. I'm smiling non-stop; I chuckle, I laugh to myself. Sometimes I'm caught jumping up and down by early-morning commuters. All they can see is my head bobbing up and down – hilarious!

I start my affirmations by saying 'good morning' to the universe, and then to my Nanny and Granddad, asking these questions every time I bounce:

- What do I believe?
- How do I want to feel at this moment?
- What is my purpose?
- What do I love?

I repeat my racing mantras out loud; I then gently review my business, making sure I am keeping it in line with my passion and purpose.

- Who are my clients?
- What do my clients want?

I know saying these words out loud can feel weird or odd. Believe me, I understand. Wait until you have to speak into a mirror – that feels odd. If you do feel intimidated or so uncomfortable you are contemplating not doing this, say them in your mind. You need only talk to yourself. Only you can answer these amazing questions.

Daily affirmations/mantras while lymphasizing

There is no generally accepted definition of mantra. Although in Sanskrit it means a sacred utterance, sound or word, some believe it to have a psychological and spiritual meaning. The literal translation is 'instrument of thought'.

Is the concept of a mantra new to you? I have used mantras ritually for training and on race days. Rhythmically using a mantra has brought me strength and inspiration when my energy dips during a race. The mantra I use is 'I am strong, I am amazing'.

I repeat in a 1-2-3 rhythm, in time with the rhythm of my running. Please enjoy using these words, until such time as you have found your own rhythm and inner voice. The results are phenomenal. In the darkest places of an Ironman challenge, I uttered these words and from these words came greatness.

Whenever I race, there are times where I say to myself, 'Why am I doing this?' 'I hate this!' 'It doesn't define me!','Nobody cares about what I achieve!' blah blah blah. This is when you want to have a tantrum, stamp your feet and shout 'I want to go home!' As an athlete, you know these times will come; it's not a question of 'will they?' it's 'when?' I must share with you my secret written word for racing. I suppose you could call it a mantra.

I prepare by writing my son's name, Jack, on the inside of my forearm. I write his name to remind me of the pain he confronts every day. You see, Jack is autistic. He is the most inspirational human I know. He challenges me, his siblings, and the whole of the universe. He would give you his last Rolo, and then smack you in the mouth for it.

The momentary, intermittent pain that racing inflicts on you is soon over. It may be intense, often unbearable, but it always ends, whereas Jack's pain is constant. He can never get away from himself. His psychological turmoil is relentless, his chronic anguish constant. His facial tics from Tourette's are painful to watch, never mind the lip cuts he creates and the soreness of his facial muscles. His internal pain is never-ending.

Embrace the power of the word, the word said internally at first and then aloud to the Universe.

Daily Ritual 5: Daily importance

It's safe to say that you are bound to feel resistance when going through the 11 daily rituals. The resistance will become stronger the further you travel through this chapter. Allow it to land on you, breathe, and dance with fear.

Dancing with fear? That's like saying 'friendly fire' or 'pleasurable pain'. As I am informed by Noos, my daughter, this is called an oxymoron. Its words contradict each other.

'Dancing with fear' is not contradictory. It's an action. It's a conscious thought process. Dancing with fear creates fun, laughter, and a flow of energy that generates momentum. Being fearless goes against our primal instinct of 'fight or flight'. Going against the flow (the words alone create feelings of resistance) consumes your energy.

Being fearful also consumes your energy. It blocks emotion. It stops you from moving towards your dreams. It keeps you from the most crucial element in gaining any result: action. Being fearful paralyses you..

Ask yourself the greatest question:

'How do I feel ?' Complete it with 'How do I feel about dancing with fear?'

This always makes me smile. It's a pattern interrupter. It confuses you. You know that the word fear is nothing to smile about. But creating an oxymoron can generate a desire to engage with it.

'I want to dance with fear'; 'I can dance with fear'.

It makes it fun; it disrupts your thoughts, creating emotions that allow you to move towards your dreams.

I can feel you now; I can hear you now.

'I want to dance with fear'; 'I can dance with fear'.

Have you ever questioned what is important to you? More importantly, what is important to you on a daily basis?

ACTION

Take five minutes to ask yourself:

'What is important to me on a daily basis?'

Write the wisdom you are sharing in your journal; it is gold dust. It needs to get into your nervous system and deeper into your cellular structure. You must feel the importance in every cell.

Here are my daily 'importances' to support you in your thoughts.

1. I must exercise/open my body to feed my soul
2. I must put goodness into my body with organic food
3. I must write for 1 hour every day.
4. I must meditate for 20 minutes.
5. I must read a book for 1 hour.

These importances that I have identified feed my soul and nourish my body so that I can be my daily best. Being my daily best is a must for me, my family, my friends and for the wonderful clients that I support every day. Being my daily best builds the foundations needed for my higher purpose: sharing knowledge and supporting people to believe in their health. It makes sense to me first to feed myself with love, respect and goodness, then – and only then – am I equipped to travel along my extraordinary pathway.

Notice that none of the above is urgent. What does urgent mean to you? To me, urgent has to be life-threatening. Urgent is always someone else's feeling, not mine. What is the difference between something being urgent and something being important? Is anything in your day so urgent that you should stop doing what is important to you, to your life's purpose, to your vision, to your thoughts of success, or to your values and beliefs? In a word, *no!*

Get ready to rage inwardly. Emails are other people's urgencies. Stop fulfilling others' urgencies at the expense of your daily importances. Just stop and breathe. How often do you check emails? Once or twice a day? Hourly? Even worse, every 15 minutes? Just stop.

Start to think of a daily strategy to allow these rituals into your life. Unless these rituals become part of your life, your resistance will stop you from growing into wisdom. You can have all the knowledge and think you are wise, but you have to put wisdom, into practice. You cannot know wisdom; you can only be wisdom.

ACTION

Time this action. It should take no longer than 5 minutes.

Write a list in your journal of five daily essential/important activities that you must do to be your daily best. Remind yourself this is not urgent stuff, but it's what must be done to keep you to your life's purpose.

Knowing what is consistently important to you will ignite your passion every day.

Daily Ritual 6: Fasted movement/exercise

No Extra Time Training (NETT)

Keeping moving throughout the day, outdoors, is a must. It seems ludicrous even to have to say this, but because of the way society has evolved, walking has become a thing of the past. When I suggest exercise to successful, busy, people, time is the biggest excuse. The usual reply to me 'It's all right for you, you've always exercised', or 'It's alright for you, you like getting up early'. I could give you an endless list of It's alright for you's.

My clients include busy, successful, women who travel the globe, which makes working out/exercising impossible. I needed to create an effective method of movement using the most effective piece of equipment you have: your body and its weight.

Not only can NETT provide you with an investment in your future mobility, it turns the fat switch on: you will become a fat-burning machine. The results always astound me.

NETT consists of two methods, fasted walking or high-intensity interval training (HIIT). Neither method needs a gym, and both can accommodate travel.

At a workshop I attended years ago, a highly acclaimed speaker gave me a jolt with these words: 'If you don't have 10 minutes to give to your body, you don't have a life.' Harsh but true. Everyone can establish daily disciplines in their lives.

How does the word 'discipline' make you feel? For me, the word 'discipline' creates a force within me. It allows my body to know that I have returned to my purpose. Choosing discipline will enable you to stay on your path rather than be wooed by distraction. Discipline is challenging. Discipline can at times be painful, both physically and emotionally. Discipline is needed to do and go where others would stop and settle for less.

Being an athlete requires you to have discipline in your life. You know where you are and where you are heading. Knowing that the challenges you face can be endured keeps you focused and your self-belief alive.

A dear friend once told me that a challenge is only a challenge if you have less than a 50% chance of succeeding. That made me smile. Then I asked myself, 'Knowing that the chance of failure is so high, would I begin such a challenge?' The answer is only ever 'yes'.

Your quest, your challenge is to put your blessed body against the 'gods of time', and create daily disciplines that keep you focused on peak energy performance every day. Everyone should invest in a movement/fitness regime.

It is your duty to embrace movement and health. It should never be a choice. But the busier the universe is gets the more removed from the truth this is. It appears that human beings are beginning to view health as optional. This is is nonsensical.

We, as a species, have never been so unwell or so overweight. Human fertility is on the decline, along with our mobility. We ignore our bodies' need for water and fresh seasonal foods. It is safe to say that our stressful, busy, quick-fix behaviours, sedentary life and processed foods can put up their hands and take the blame.

Simple, quick, effective movements can be prescribed to start you on your journey back to efficient energy. And if your food is boxed or in a wrapper, ask yourself. 'Where would I find this growing?' You will get to a stage where it is unthinkable not to do your daily NETT. It would be like someone suggesting breathing without oxygen: unfathomable.

NETT is super-simple. All you need is you, a wild imagination and the ability to grunt and groan!

Fasted Walking/exercise

Fasted walking is a beautiful place to begin your journey of moving into you.

Start from where you are today. NETT is not only for people who are sporty. It is inclusive. Wherever you are, that's where you start from.

I have women asking me to train them for a marathon. They have never run, but have tried, and can accomplish, 60 seconds of running. They go and achieve their dreams: marathon, tick. And all with the life approach system: dreams, devotion, determination and discipline.

Walking is kind to the body. It makes a minimal impact and generates wonderful emotions. Movement is the key to creating powerful emotions. If 20 minutes of walking brings fear and failure into your thoughts, breathe and know that this is a true challenge. Accept the challenge, and prepare for greatness.

At the beginning of any challenge, the goal is to achieve something. If 20 minutes is out of the question, start with a more achievable time. The structure is still the same; the discipline is still the same: you are creating rituals of behaviour. These are the foundations of your energy efficiency. The numbers are irrelevant, the actions are a must.

'Fasted'? What does that mean? No, it doesn't mean walking very, very, very fast. What I mean is that you must move or exercise before you have eaten.

'Fasted' exercise in its true sense is movement/exercise taken during a period of time in which the insulin levels in your body are low. The body is no longer processing food or absorbing it; this is a fasted state.

Again, we are manipulating the hormones at a cellular level to produce efficient energy, keeping the cells clean and lean. 'Clean and lean' is an approach to decision-making while you are focused on producing efficient cellular energy. It's not just about nutrition/diet or detoxing the body. It's about choosing to make the best decision for yourself at that moment, based on what you choose to think about yourself and your environment:

- The relationships you choose to keep or let go of.
- The career/job you choose to spend your time at.
- The words that you use every day to yourself/your family/other people.
- The movement you choose to put your body through every day.
- The food you choose to eat and feed your family with.

Can you see the common denominator in the concept of 'clean and lean'? It relates both to you and to the decisions you make about the choices you find yourself with.

- Keeping the mind clean of dirty words that clog up your cells = HIGH ENERGY
- Keeping the body clean of toxins from processed food and drink = HIGH ENERGY
- Keeping the body clean of sedentary living/lack of movement = HIGH ENERGY
- Keeping the environment clean of negative relationships = HIGH ENERGY

Keep your thoughts LEAN
Keep your environment LEAN
Keep your body LEAN

Here is your passport to an explosion of energy, every single day.

ACTION

Fasted walking/exercise

Begin today, at the start of your morning. Start from where you are today. You are aiming for 20 minutes.

Begin by observing how your foot strikes on the ground.

Do you land your heel first, or mid-foot? How does the movement feel as the power from your foot strike accelerates up through the body? Are you able to keep the beautiful posture described in Chapter 8? The body should feel centred throughout the forward motion.

Keep the foot strike underneath your body. Your stride should fall underneath you. Making your stride longer will encourage heel striking, which is very normal with today's footwear, but it can cause stress through lower body joints. Keep centred throughout your walk.

Don't be tempted to sacrifice posture and the correct form of motion for speed. Speed can easily be introduced once your posture and the correct form of motion are embedded in your nervous system.

ACTION

Progressing fasted walking

Now you have begun to incorporate fasted walking into your day, you are able to adapt this practice.

Start with walking, focusing on form. After 5 minutes of mindful walking, increase your speed.

You will notice your body adapting. You have added a stimulus – exercise – for the body to respond to and grow into. The increase in speed prevents the body from 'plateau-ing', which is when you continue to do the same thing but the body has got used to the exercise, so it no longer has as great an impact. This means another type of stimulus is needed for growth to continue, in this case, increasing the speed.

Variable speeds shock the body, keeping it guessing. Increase the speed for 2 minutes, and then pull back for 30–60 seconds. It is vital for you to listen to your body's feedback. If you need nearer 60 seconds than 30 to recover, then take the full allocation of time. Recovery will not bring you right back to your original state. You should feel ready to go again, with a hint of challenge looming.

Repeat this pattern for 10 minutes: 2 minutes of high-speed walking, followed by 30–60 seconds at a reduced speed. You should feel as you did the end of the first 5 minutes, before you started the high-speed walk.

Once the 10-minute interval walk is complete, you will be 15 minutes into your 20-minute walk. Return to your steady, settled speed for the remaining 5 minutes.

You are now on your way to utilizing your fat stores for fuel. This creates a lean body that produces efficient cellular energy.

High intensity interval training (HIIT)

This method is super-effective in turning the body's fat switch on. It encourages the body to use its stores of fat as fuel. Let me explain.

For optimum health the body must be clean and lean, detoxified daily. A lean body has a lower fat composition. Toxins are stored in the fat in your body. The leaner we are the fewer toxins we store, creating energy in abundance.

Toxins are inescapable in our society. They are in our hair products, body washes, shower water, tap water, processed foods, meats and the soil our non-organic food is grown in. I'll stop here – the list is endless.

Every day you should be asking yourself, 'What toxins does this product contain?' You always have a choice, what you drink and what you eat. One of my all-time favourite films, *Dangerous Minds* starring Michelle Pfeiffer, captures the essence of choice. 'It may not be a choice you like, but it is a choice.'

Sometimes you have to make the best decision you can from equally unattractive options.

A great example of this is a question I am asked every day: 'Which is better for me: Fat Coke or Diet Coke?' This may not be the choice you want, but which is best decision to make out of the choice that you find yourself with? This choice is not in alignment with health or vitality but a choice that people may find themselves in, especially our children. Water seems to be a blind choice.

Please be kind to yourself. You can only do your best with the choice that you see in front of you.

HIIT training is high intensity intervals of exertion for a very short period of time, followed by low to moderate intensity exertion for an even shorter recovery time.

There are many styles of HIIT training. Tabata is a great example: intense, all-out movement for anything from 20 seconds, with 10 seconds recovery, repeated for 20 minutes, up to 40–50 seconds of giving it your all, followed by 10–20 seconds recovery. You titrate the workout phases and rest phases to your current capabilities.

You can see how vital it is to understand yourself and your body, to know exactly where you are and where you are going. And always start with the end in mind; that is true of any form of exercise. It must be achievable.

HIIT training has so many benefits:

1. Burns more fat in less time
2. Ideal for time poor people (that's everyone, then).
3. Better results than steady cardio exercise, thanks to EPOC. (Excess Post Exercise Consumption: a period of 16–24 hours post-exercise recovery to re-oxygenate the depleted muscles. Build oxygen stores back up in the body takes up more energy, using stored fat as fuel.
4. Can be done at home, so quicker, and no need to travel to the gym.
5. Stimulates growth hormone. This depletes over time, so it's all about how we can we manipulate our hormones to produce our desired outcome.
6. It's short, sharp, intense – then over and done with.
7. Good for blood pressure, cholesterol profiles, insulin levels and cardiovascular health (The American College of Sports Science).
8. Minimal equipment needed.
9. Supports control of blood sugar.

And there are many more benefits related to this style of movement. Practise this form of exercise once to four times a week. Again, know yourself, your starting point; listen to your body and exercise according to your level.

You are building your body up, not breaking it down.

ACTION

A new routine always needs to be simple, repetitive and achievable. You have to want to do it again after the first go.

Take five exercises, simple exercise that you are familiar with. Here are some of the most loved and popular ones.

- Press-ups
- Burpees
- Jumping Jacks
- Squats with variations
- Lunges with variations
- Running up stairs
- Massive jump onto a step/stair
- Plank and variations (e.g. walking into it)
- Sit-ups/Curl-ups
- Handstands
- Tuck jumps
- Sprinting on the spot
- Get creative.

Now for the timings.

Remember that you must make your exercise goal achievable at the beginning of practising this ritual.

Listen to your body and adjust the timings according to your capabilities.

A great place to start is with 40 seconds 'all out' and 20 seconds of active rest.

You can always build on this to support your goal. Always make it achievable at the beginning.

Become playful with the timings:

- 40 seconds all out, 20 seconds active rest
- 50 seconds all out, 10 seconds active rest
- 55 seconds all out, 5 seconds active rest
- 1 minute all out, NO REST, straight onto the next exercise.

Active rest could entail a gentle walk around the room, keeping the heart rate elevated, But NO standing still.

You need to keep your blood flowing around the body, helping the blood flow in the legs to return to the heart. If you just stood still you would get 'blood pooling', so it's super-important to keep moving the legs gently. (That doesn't mean you can get super-creative/cheeky and lie on the floor with your legs up in the air.)

Start with a gentle warm-up: running on the spot or skipping for 2 – 3 minutes.

It is vital to prepare the body for exercise.(If you were time rich, you could mix it up: do the fasted walk, followed immediately by ten minutes of HIIT. This takes up 30 minutes of your day.)

Your goal is a total of 10 minutes. Keep it simple. You could repeat one exercise five times or do five in sequence to make up your 10 minutes.

Once you have completed your HIIT, gently walk around, recover, then it is on to the next part of your day: Daily Ritual 7, opening up the body.

Daily Ritual 7: Body opening

Opening your body up in the morning prepares you for creativity throughout the day. There are multiple ways of opening up the body to the energy flow of the universe, to yourself, to your thoughts, your dreams, and to others. Of creating space for energy to flow. Ask yourself this question, 'How can I become welcoming to opportunity if I feel closed inside?'

ACTION

Inside the spring

Whether you are skilled in visualization or not, I'm sure you can imagine how it would feel to be inside a tightly coiled spring. We are all at different levels of body awareness, but feel it we do, so have a go at this visualization.

- Close your eyes.
- Visualize yourself in the middle of a tightly coiled spring.

- How does it feel?
- Transfer this feeling into imagining that your body is the tightly coiled spring
- Make a fist with your hand (any hand, preferably yours!)
- Make it tight, tighter, tighter again.
- Keep the pressure in the fist.
- Keep squeezing, and squeezing, and squeezing.
- Keep on squeezing.
- You should have had enough by now: it's uncomfortable, it's painful, it goes numb after a while.
- Keep squeezing.
- Observe your thoughts.
- Observe the way this exercise makes you feel.
- Observe the pain. Do you feel any pain?
- Observe the pain. Does the pain stimulus change?
- Observe your breathing.
- Observe your body language: are you pacing around while squeezing your hand?

Transfer your findings to the coiled spring. You can feel the energy it takes to keep the force so tightly packed within the spring. It takes a huge amount of energy to keep in this one intense space, energy that you cannot afford to expend elsewhere.

When I do this exercise it always makes me feel absolutely fatigued. It affects my breathing, my inner sense of being. My chest feels tight; my breathing becomes shallow and short. I feel nervousness take over my body. I don't enjoy feeling this way. It creates a sense of 'I can't'. It's exhausting living in this limited space. This is not where I want to live every day.

Opening up the body allows energy to flow. Opening your body will open your thoughts. It certainly makes me smile, opens up my breath. I can feel my cells vibrating with energy and excitement. This is a place I choose to be in every day.

Opening the body always follows exercise or movement. There are so many options available to you. It's super-important that you listen to your body and choose the option that you believe opens your body.

I have chosen three alternative methods that I am committed to and practice as part of my life of movement. I share them with you to inspire you to begin your search to find what is right for you.

What makes you feel amazing? What makes you want to spend time there?

ACTION

What would enable you to open up your body? Write your thoughts in your journal, but in a different colour from your other entries. You will be returning to these thoughts.

'Know thy self.'

When you are introducing any new technique to your body, you should always follow the same protocol.

1. Listen to your body.
2. Start from where you are today, not from what you used to be able to achieve.
3. Move into a challenged position, towards discomfort, but not pain.
4. Stop if you feel pain.
5. Build up your every day, don't break it down. You must love your body.

The Five Tibetan Rites: the 'Fountain of Youth'

Although these rituals have several titles, they all originate from five exercises to be practised daily, coordinating the breath with movement. There is a sixth exercise with many theories behind it. Sounds mystical? I will introduce the sixth ritual and you can choose whether it is suitable for your body.

These movement sequences are reputed to be over 2,500 years old. They were brought to the western world by a retired British Army officer, Colonel Bradford. This is a pen name, though, for the booklet entitled *'Ancient Secret of the Fountain of Youth* was actually written by Peter Kelder, who melded fact and fiction in sharing these magical ancient rites. It is said that a retired gentleman, 'Colonel Bradford', a frail old man with a terrific sense of wonder from his travels, sat down next to Peter Kelder in a park. They went on to become great friends, sharing stories of their experiences in the east.

While travelling in the Himalayas, the Colonel found a monastery, which, according to legend, held the ancient secrets to youth and rejuvenation.

Colonel Bradford was known by the lamas as 'The Ancient One', as everyone else around him had a youthful appearance. During his stay he was given full details about the 'Fountain of Youth.'

According to Kelder's book, ill health is caused by our energy centres – chakras – being blocked or unbalanced. The word 'chakra' is derived from the Sanskrit language and means 'wheel', translated literally from Hindi as 'wheel of spinning energy'. This gives us a wonderful visual as to the way energy moves around the body, in a vortex, a powerhouse, of energy. The vision it creates is a centred power circling, swirling, with an even force within it.

There are many chakras in the body that play a vital role in our physiology and conscious thought processes.

Location of chakras

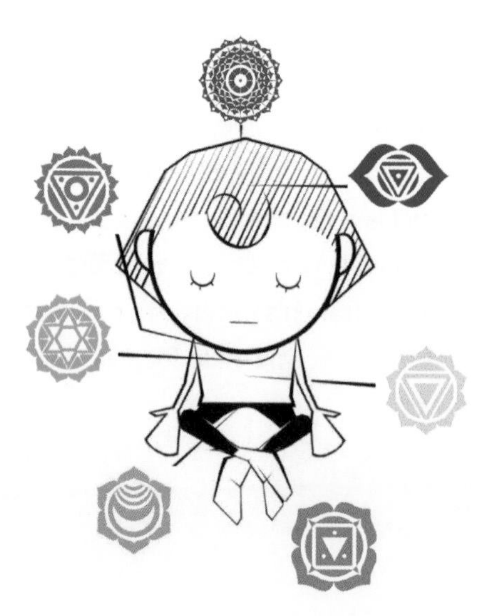

Root Chakra

Functions: Safety, grounding, right to live

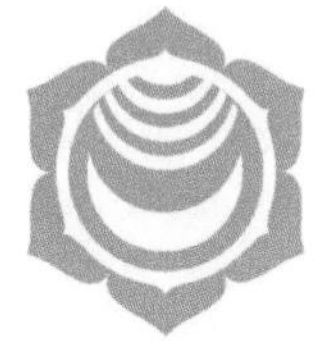

Sacral Chakra

Functions: Emotions, creativity, sexuality

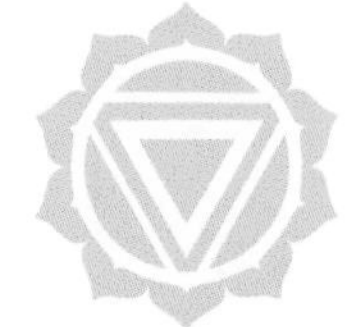

Solar Plexus Chakra

Functions: Will, social self, power

Heart Chakra

Functions: Compassion, love, integration

Throat Chakra

Function: Personal truth, etheric, expression

Third Eye Chakra

Functions: Extrasensory perception, intuition, inspiration

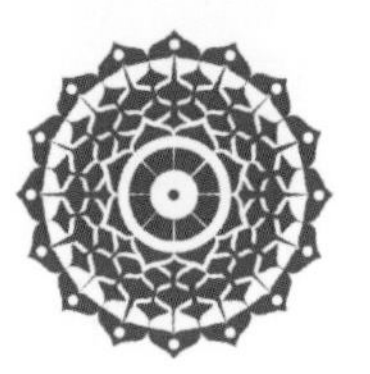

Crown Chakra

Functions: Wisdom, transcendence, universality

There are seven main chakras. As a Pilates teacher, I know that alignment of the spine is fundamental to movement. It makes complete sense to align your physiology with your energy centers, thus balancing your external structure with your internal physiology. Feeling balanced creates power; power over yourself. The word 'centred' comes to the forefront. When you are centred, balanced, you feel strong, able to be successful in your day. Aligning your energy, centring your body, is a beautiful ritual to give yourself every day.

This is the purpose of the 'Five Tibetan Rites'.

The movements/exercises are to be part of your daily movement for your body. These movements will ignite your internal strength, boost your energy and create a mindset of total belief in yourself. They are called the 'Fountain of Youth' because when you feel amazing, able to move with strength and ease, it creates an ageless mindset. You don't even think of age as a factor. It does not affect your choices or the decisions you make. You feel you can do whatever you choose to do. It is non-restrictive.

Being able to do what you choose in your life with no limits or restrictions from your body – isn't that optimum health? This was the response I got when I put young people into focus groups together. I spoke to over 100 young people aged 13 to 18, asking them to share their views on what they believed optimum health looked like. They were from different social groups, geographical areas and educational backgrounds, but they all agreed that 'To have health, optimum health, is to have no restrictions from your body when you want to do something.'

Where in our lives did we lose this understanding? When did we choose to ignore the opportunities to invest our bodies with greatness every day? To be too busy to factor in daily movement?

Become an artist. Every day with these movements, begin to create an ageless mind and body. Become free in your movements. Become free in your energy. Become free in your thoughts.

Practising every day encourages the chakras to perform at optimum energy, creating a balance of thoughts and mood, of hormones throughout the body, and harmony within you. You know the feeling you get during your day, the nervousness cellular shake when you are busy being busy? Then from this peak state you drop with a tremendous thud, unable to pick yourself up as you haven't the energy left. Living in this 'peaks and troughs' state is exhausting. You think you are performing with amazing results, but it takes its toll on your relationships and, more importantly, on your love for yourself. These feelings, these thoughts, will stop. I'm excited for you. I'm smiling at the prospect of the daily joy you are about to release into your life. Let these words land on you: daily joy. Daily!

Tibetan Rite 1

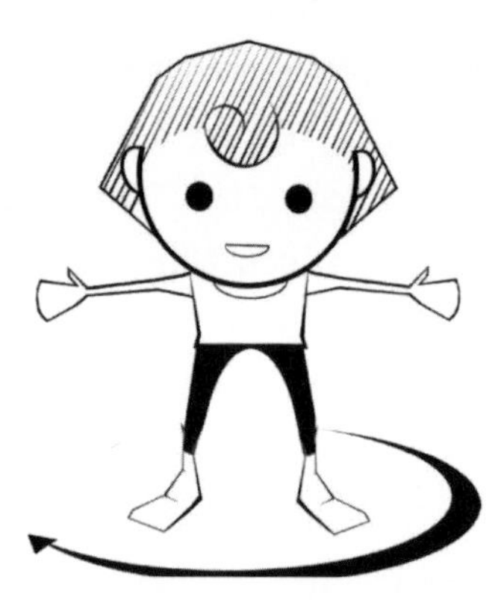

- Stand tall with your shoulders, hips and ankles in alignment. Have your arms stretched out to the sides and your shoulders are drawn down away from your ears.
- Holding the arms in this position, begin to turn in a clockwise direction, turning the feet on the spot and allowing the head to lead or follow the move.
- Repeat 21 times – no more than 21 repetitions are needed.

I have researched the reasoning behind only turning clockwise and the number repetitions, and I can't I find a convincing explanation. But, I am going with it: the results you achieve are the answers to the 'why's.

When you begin this rite, it can make you dizzy. Work with the body you find yourself with today. Start with three to five repetitions and build from where you are today. Always build, never break. You are building confidence in your movements and in yourself. I have had clients who have felt obsessively that they 'must complete all the repetitions' and have felt so sick throughout the rest of the Rites that they have stopped them halfway through; then decided not to incorporate the Rites into their life. Start from where you are today: love every breath and movement you are giving yourself; trust in the movements and watch magic happen.

Tibetan Rite 2

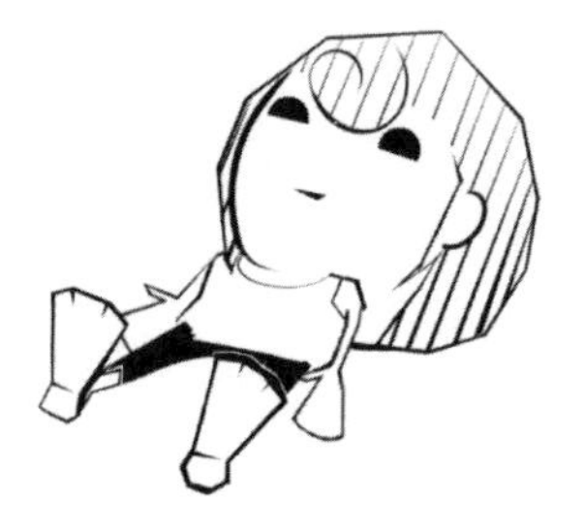

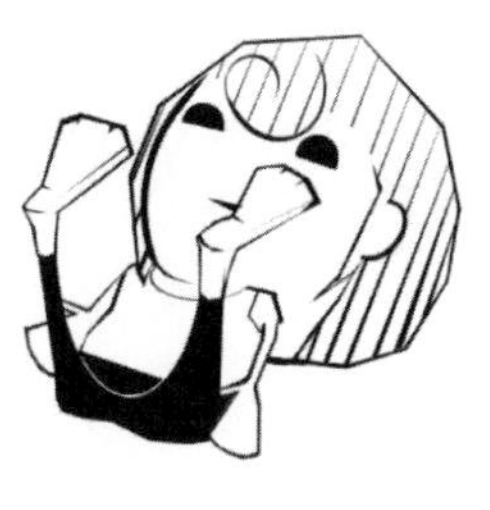

- Lie on the floor with your legs fully lengthened.
- Place the hands palm down and allow the body to relax onto the floor or mat.
- As you inhale (breathe in), raise your outstretched legs and head simultaneously.

- Take the legs past the 90-degree angle over the head. The back will imprint into the mat.
- Raise your head, tucking your chin into your chest. Move with ease and purpose – no sticky movement. The toes are pointed to the ceiling (plantar flexion).
- As you lower the lengthened legs and bring your head back to the starting position, exhale (breathe out).

Then repeat, to a maximum of 21 repetitions.

This move should never cause pain. If it does, adapt the move. No adaptations to the moves have been documented, which means these exercises may not be very inclusive. But I have taught the Tibetan Rites to hundreds of clients and have developed adaptations to the moves. These enable everyone to incorporate the Tibetan Rites into their daily lives.

If this move causes you pain or you do not feel able to lift your outstretched legs, follow these adaptations. Begin in the starting position: the legs should be bent, with the soles of the feet on the floor. Here are two options.

Option 1

- Keep both legs bent at the knees at a 90° angle and lift them both at the same time.
- As you lengthen the legs up over your head, raise your head and shoulders to the position described above.
- Point your feet to the ceiling (plantar flexion).
- Lower the legs in exactly the same way as lifting, back to the starting position.

- Continue to breathe in as you raise the legs, and out as you lower them.

Do as many as you can manage, up to a maximum of 21 repetitions – pain free.

Option 2

- In your starting position, with the soles of the feet on the floor (semi-supine position), lift one leg up to a 90angle at the knee, then lift the second leg off to join it.
- From this position, with the shins parallel to the floor, lengthen both legs out and raise the head and shoulders.
- Lower the legs in exactly the same way as you lifted them, back to the starting position. Continue to breathe in as you raise the legs, and out as you lower them.

Do as many as you can manage, up to a maximum of 21 repetitions – pain free.

Peter Kelder quotes a story told by Colonel Bradford in his book *The Eye of Revelation.*

When the Colonel was in the Tibetan monastery, one of the lamas told him that he was unable to lift both legs up when he began the Rites. He was too weak, he felt too old. But he started to lift his legs little by little, not completing the actual move, but adapting it to what he could do at that moment.

With belief and time, he was able to move with purpose and ease through the complete sequence. The Colonel marveled at the lama, as he was the picture of health and youth.

First, ask yourself, 'How do I feel at this moment?' Adapt the move to *you*. Believe, and invest your time in beautiful movement.

Tibetan Rite 3

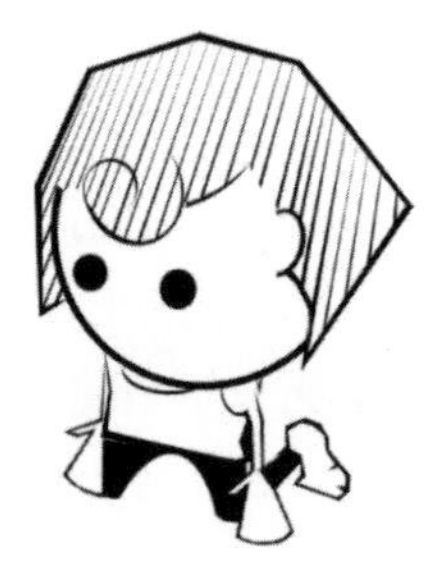

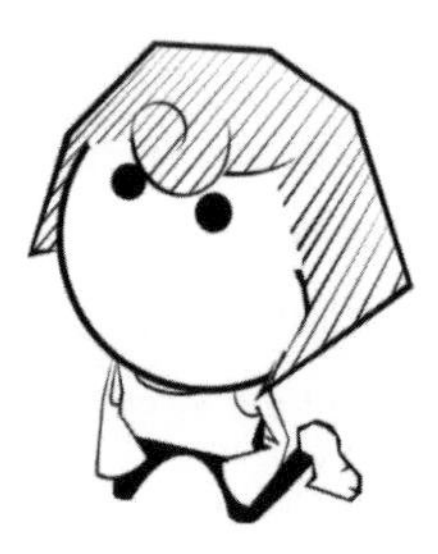

- Start in a kneeling position, with the toes/balls of your feet anchoring you to the floor.
- Place your hands just under the buttocks/gluteus maximus, at the tops of the thighs.
- Exhale and begin to bend forward gently at the waist, bringing the chin towards the chest, and rolling the shoulders gently forward.
- Inhale, bring the face up towards the ceiling, with the throat open/lengthened and the back creating an arch.
- Lean back as far as possible, allowing the arms and hands to support you. Your toes will prevent you from falling backwards.
- Inhale, return your chin towards your chest.

Do not move into pain; work with the body you find yourself in at this moment. Repeat, up to 21 repetitions. Build your body daily, don't break it.

To adapt the move, work within your body's ability. Listen to your body and identify what feels challenging but not painful. When beginning on this move be kind to yourself. Do not lean back so far that your back twinges or you cause an injury to your body. Your focus is always on building the body, not breaking it in a moment of self-competitiveness.

Tibetan Rite 4

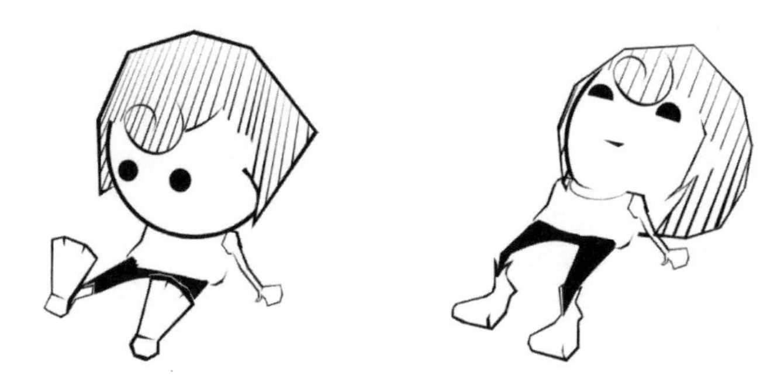

- Sit tall into your spine, with your hands directly alongside your hips and your legs lengthened out in front of you, feet flexed towards your shins (dorsi-flexion).
- The chin rests on the chest, lengthening the back of the neck.
- The head leads the move, as your face tilts towards the ceiling and the back of the neck shortens. (You may hear all sorts of noises: breathe into the move).
- At the same time, shift your weight onto your hands to support you as you lift your body. The knees bend at 90° and the soles of the feet have full contact with the floor.

- Inhale as you lift your hips till they are parallel to the floor. You will feel open at the hips, tight in the buttocks/gluteus maximus, and the shoulders feel open at the front from the breastbone to the shoulder joint.
- Exhale, lowering yourself back to your seated starting position.

This is a super-powerful, open move. Repeat, to maximum of 21 repetitions. Listen to your body. Start from where you are today, not from where you think you should be or from what you used to be able to do.

Adaptations for Rite 4

If your body is laughing at you, saying 'there is no way I can do that', bring your hips up as high as you can. Do not move into pain. Your wrists may be screaming 'What are you doing to me?' Ask yourself how often you bear weight on your wrists when they are bent at 90°. Then breathe, pause, breathe again and always be kind to yourself.

If you are unable to bear weight on your shoulders, try this:

- Lie on your back on the floor, with soles of your feet in contact with the floor.
- Balance the weight evenly through the feet: big toe, little toe, outside of the heel, inside of the heel.
- Keeping your shoulders on the floor, gently lift the hips towards the ceiling, inhaling as you do so.
- The weight shifts to the shoulders, and the chin moves towards the chest as the back of the neck lengthens.
- Exhale as you lower back down to your starting position.

- Continue to inhale and lift, pause and exhale and lower, to a maximum of 21 repetitions or your body's capability.

Build and grow every day.

Tibetan Rite 5

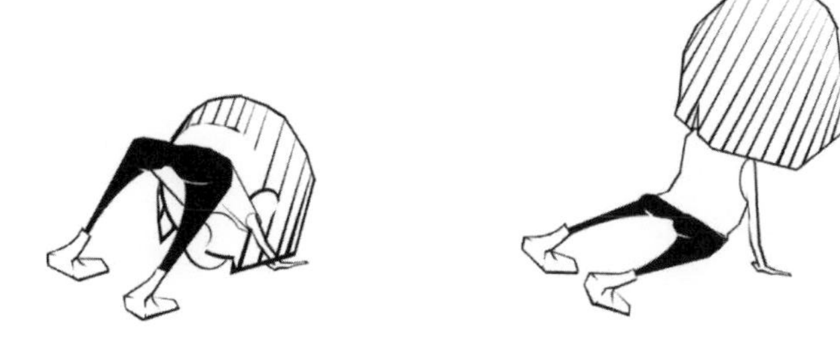

This is a super-powerful move that gives you the opportunity to progress your breathing techniques and to pause within the move.

- Start in a press-up/plank position, with your weight distributed equally through your hands and feet. Your wrists, elbows and shoulders should be aligned, and your weight distributed equally between your hands (fingers splayed) and your toes.
- Push the body through the hips upwards towards the ceiling, into an inverted 'V' shape. Allow the head to relax, push back into the shoulders, with your weight evenly distributed between your hands and your feet. You should try to bring your heels to the floor, stretching the backs of your legs.
- From this position, shift your weight forward, lowering the body parallel to the floor, arching the back, keeping the legs active and lengthened, and keeping the arms and legs straight.

- Your face is tilted towards the ceiling, lengthened under the chin and shortened at the back of the neck.
- The hands and feet remain on the floor for the entire move, but the rest of the body remains suspended throughout.
- Energy should flow throughout this move. You should leading from your centre, lifting up through the pelvis.

(I adore this move. I feel open, mobile, connected to myself within my body. I feel strong, able to be my daily best.)

Repeat the move, up to maximum of 21 repetitions. Work with the body you find yourself in today.

Adaptations for Rite 5

If you have shoulder injuries or are unable to bear much weight on your arms , please give yourself this gift:do not move into pain.

Adaptation 1

This is exactly the same movement, but on bent arms.

- Keep your elbows directly under your shoulders, and your hands and forearms in contact with the floor/mat, with your weight evenly distributed.
- Your bottom is in the air, tailbone pointing to the sky, your knees are under your hips, and the front of the feet is in contact with the floor.
- From your centre, move the hips up to the ceiling/sky, dropping the heels.

- Shift the weight forward; dropping your head back and tilting the face towards the ceiling.

Continue repeating the move, up to 21 repetitions.

Adaptation 2

If you are unable to bear weight through your shoulders and arms, use this adaptation.

- Adopt the starting position as in Adaptation1.
- Initiate the move from your centre, breathe out (exhale) and lengthen one leg away from the body, keeping the foot in contact with the floor.
- As you breathe in (inhale), draw the leg back in 'from whence it came.' Keep the foot in contact with the floor throughout the move.
- Use your breath to create a rhythm for the movement.
- After each leg lengthening, remain in the centred position and tilt your face towards the ceiling, lengthening the front of the neck and shortening the back of it. The spine creates a curve: face up to the sky, tailbone up to the sky, and the spine dipped and shortened in the middle.

Do not move into pain. Repeat the move, to a maximum of 21 repetitions. Listen to your body.

After completing the Five Rites, allow your body to settle. Either sit on the floor/mat, with your body upright, aligning the hips, shoulder and the head on a lengthened neck, allowing the breath to return to its pre-exercise state; or you can stand, grounded weight even through the feet, abdominals engaged, pelvic floor connected, your ribcage connected not flaring, with your shoulders naturally falling forward, and 'restack' your head. Feel strong, lengthened and grounded into the earth, and breathe. You may close your eyes to challenge your centre. And breathe, feeling powerful with each breath. As you breathe in, use the mantra 'open'. As you breathe out, use the mantra 'release'.

Tibetan Rite 6: 'Elixir of Life'

'But you said there were Five Rites!'

Peter Kelder insists that this is an extension practice, only to be attempted once the Five Rites have been incorporated into your life with good results. In Kelder's writings, the Colonel explains that this progressive move/rite is for one who has 'excess procreative energy'. Christopher S. Kilham describes the sixth rite as an accompaniment to the main sequence.

Its historical purpose is for transmuting sexual energy upwards, through the energy chakras, creating powerful energy, rather than downwards, causing agitation, blocked emotions and exhaustion.

The Colonel suggests anyone who feels a powerful reproductive urge should complete the sixth rite. According to Peter Kelder's understanding of the Tibetan Rites, they originated in a monastery where celibacy is a daily practice. For many religions/spiritual practices, sexual activity hinders the attainment of enlightenment. According to the Colonel, when this sexual energy moves downwards, it produces an 'average man', whereas by moving the energy upwards, towards enlightenment, you create a strong, powerful, magnetized 'superman'. To you transform into a 'superman' you draw on the true 'Elixir of Life'. He suggests that the average man is only interested in material things, and therefore need only practise the Five Rites. The man who desires enlightenment should make a clean start, which will lead him to living a 'superlife'. This was written in 1938–1939; do not allow the language to create a barrier. Merely open your thoughts to increasing your knowledge and learn from the scriptures.

I share this knowledge with you hoping not to generate resistance, but with the intention of supporting you to develop your own practice. To be sexual and sensual creates energy that is truly wonderful. Choose wisely.

Practising this rite is valuable in developing strength within the second chakra, in enhancing your energy within relationships. It has been suggested it heightens your sexual experiences, giving you strength and control during sex. You may thank me later for sharing this with you.

- Stand in your starting position, grounded, in beautiful alignment with your weight evenly distributed.
- Breathe in deeply through the nose, then allow a controlled exhale through the mouth. Settle the breath and allow your thoughts to smile.
- Breathe out, releasing every inch of breath; and engage your abdominals, pulling them in tight.
- As you breathe out, bend forward, moving only from the hips. The spine does not move. Place your hands on your knees. Continue to release as much air from the lungs as possible at this moment.
- From this position, hold/pause the breath and return to the standing position.

- Place your hands on your hips and press down on them. Continue to hold/pause the breath. Remain connected, with shoulders lowered away from the ears, abdominals engaged.
- Hold this position until you feel you *must* breathe. Control the breath, breathing through the nose with an even flow of energy.
- Release the breath through your mouth and relax your arms, allowing them to fall by your side.
- Take recovery breaths and return to your normal breath pattern.

This is one repetition. A total of three repetitions is required to balance the most powerful downward energy. This allows the energy to move upwards through the energy systems.

The Colonel makes it very clear in Peter Kelder's book that the order of the Rites be respected and you should only perform this Sixth Rite when you have become accomplished at the Five Rites; full power must be achieved before practising this sixth rite.

FAQs about the Five Rites

'How do I put these amazing movements into my day?'

Here are the answers to some of the questions I've been asked.

When is the best time to practice the Five Rites?
Either first thing in the morning (sunrise) or at the end of your day (sunset).This is the best-case scenario, if you are able to manipulate your day. In any case, they should be practised twice daily, morning and evening.

It is essential that you build them into your day, however you manage it. Always begin a new action with a feeling of moving freely into the ritual rather than allowing a resistance that moves you away from the action to develop. Invest in the Five Rites whenever you can create the space within your day. I am prescriptive with my words: hear these words, breathe, and let them land on you.

You create the space in your life. I did not say 'time'. Time is the same for all of us. What's different is what you choose to do with the 86400 seconds that you are given every day. Do you find yourself using phrases like, 'I will try to fit them in', 'When I have the time', 'It's alright for you who can find the time', 'How am I going to find more time to fit them in'?

Just reading these words that have actually been said to me by wonderfully successful women creates tightness in my body. It feels toxic to my body. When you catch yourself saying these toxic words, *stop!* Breathe and smile.

Have faith that you are creating space to build the body you desire.

How do I prepare for the Five Rites?

No preparation needed. Create a space the length of your body and the width of your arms. The beauty of the Five Rites is that you can take them anywhere with you. Have body, will travel. No equipment needed. If you have a yoga mat or exercise mat, then be my guest. But do not use not having your mat as a reason not to do the Five Rites.

Do I need to be clean before practice?

Many yogic practices suggest being clean for practice. It prepares your practice to feel more elevated. Cleanliness is a primary criterion for divinity. This ritual of cleaning beforehand may bring you joy in adding an extra dimension to the practice. It always comes back to how something makes you feel.

Personally, I do the Five Rites after a workout. I'm hot, sweaty and love to finish my workout with returning to my centre using the Five Rites. I find that practising the Five Rites can be hot and sweaty work anyway, so I always shower afterwards.

You are creating a mindset for yourself, and yourself alone. It's personal to your thoughts and feelings – everything we do involves the state we put ourselves into.

What should I wear?

One of my clients told me a story of when she was heavily pregnant. She woke her husband up gently in the early hours of the morning after discovering that her waters had broken and labour was well established. It was her second baby and there were only two-minute gaps between strong contractions.

He leapt out of bed panic-stricken, running around the room. He stopped abruptly, went over to his clothes drawers and asked, 'What shall I wear?'

Wear what works for you, whether that be comfortably tight or loose clothing. You choose, as long as it's something that creates freedom of movement for you and is non-restrictive and cooling.

What temperature should the room be? Should it be hot?

Neither hot nor cold. The best place to practise is in a well-ventilated area. Many people practise in the same place every day, either on a mat or a rug. Hard surfaces hurt.

When I practise the Five Rites in a wide open space, outside or in the gym, the first Rite becomes more challenging, as I experience dizziness in a large open space. When I'm in my normal practice space, I feel little or no dizziness.

When should I eat, before or after practice?

The Rites are best practised fasted. First thing in the morning is wonderful, just before breakfast. If you must eat, allow 3 hours before practising the Five Rites.

If you have eaten within 3 hours, the blood flow is being directed to the digestive system and not flowing freely around the body. This can create nausea. You want to be able to focus on creating freedom of energy throughout the body.

What if I can't do all the repetitions of the exercises?

This is simple. Always keep in your thoughts that you are building the body, not breaking it.

You are investing in your body every day, small amounts, but consistently. Building each day. There may be days when you do not increase the number of repetitions, or you find you can't reach the number you reached the day before. This is not your focus. Your focus is to implement movement every day for ten minutes. This is the greatest gift you will ever give to your body.

When you invest money, you have no expectations of having large amounts of money at the beginning or even in the middle of the investment period. Your expectations expand as your investment grows in time.

Never move into pain. It is vital that every-time you begin the Five Rites you start with the body you find yourself in today, not with what you had or might have. Remember the three Bs:

- BE Honest
- BE Realistic
- BE Kind to yourself

It is the span of 10 minutes that is vital, not number of the repetitions. Once you have given your body the daily practice of the Five Rites, then your flexibility and strength will grow. Always lengthen before you strengthen.

Tweaks to progress the moves

1. The soles of your feet should have four points of contact/weight distribution: big toe, little toe, outside of the heel, and inside of the heel.
2. Use your breath to develop the move. Exhale to bend forward into flexion, inhale to move backwards into extension. Use the pause between the breaths to progress the move further.
3. Use 'the pause': slow the move down and create a pause phase within it.. This is challenging. You are creating the strongest contraction a muscle can perform: isometric contraction, which entails shortening the muscle and maintaining that shortened contraction for a period of time. This is a wonderful tweak to resistance work/strength work within the body. I use this technique in Rites 2, 4 and 5.
4. When standing in an upright position, feel the length from the soles of your feet to the crown of the head. Keep your chin

slightly down and lengthen the back of your neck, shoulders away from the ears, so posture feels strong.

Tips to have the most wonderful 10-minute experience every day

1. Put love and enjoyment into each move. Begin your love affair with your body and invest in movement every day – daily consistent movement. Smile throughout the practice. Place unwavering faith in the greatness your body is embracing.
2. Focus on movement from your centre. All the moves should start from the centre of your body. To facilitate centring, pull up on your pelvic floor (the network of muscles used to interrupt the flow wee off when you go to the toilet) and feel your abdominal muscles draw into the centre of your body. You feel strong and powerful. Focus on maintaining your centre while you move.
3. Flow within the moves. As you breathe in (inhale) say 'open' in your thoughts; as you breathe out (exhale) say 'release' within. You are beginning to use mantras as a tool to build strength within your body.

The Five Rites are a beautifully simple sequence of movements with profound effects on the body. They are quick and easy to practise on a daily basis. So if you are time-poor, space-poor or find following an exercise regime challenging to follow, please fall in love with the Five Tibetan Rites.

Practised consistently every day, the Five Rites produce these benefits:

- A significant increase in energy – more the endurance type of energy
- Feeling calmer and less stressed
- Greater mental clarity, with stronger focus brighter
- Feeling stronger, more flexible, and more agile
- Better sleep, with enhanced dreams
- Lifts mood and improves wellbeing, tackling depression and
- Becoming more centred and at peace
- Improved posture.
- Greater abdominal strength—creating a strong foundation for your activities of daily living.
- Improved digestion and cleansing of the body
- Support for an easier menopause
- Alleviating the symptoms of menstruation
- Enhancing your sensual feelings
- Increased libido

The Shaolin Workout: Sifu Shi Yan Ming

The Shaolin Workout is a more intense daily movement regime, but with remarkable results. If you are seeking more freedom for your body and want to invest in a more complex process, you will embrace this daily workout.

This is a 28-day transformation programme, focused on stretching the body and mind. This workout requires no equipment, just you and your thoughts. It can be performed in your home, even in small spaces. You don't need a mirror to check your position when stretching, as it is said, 'your body knows when it is doing it correctly'. Mirrors can be a distraction from feeling the position.

Based on the fundamentals of kung-fu, Shaolin is a day-by-day exercise programme divided into four 1-week blocks. The kung-fu warrior draws powers from lightness, speed and clarity of mind, making decisions quickly and naturally, not becoming stagnant and over-analyzing. Introducing daily meditations brings clarity, balance and harmony, thus improving your daily life by giving you more energy and vitality.

It trains your entire body to have fast-acting, long muscles, building strength through speed and agility. It extends your body, mind and spirit, infusing your activities of daily living with confidence and a sense of 'beautiful calm'.

Daily practice of this workout builds your love of training your body. The more you move, the more you will want to train and the more your love of moving your body will grow. Purposeful daily repetition of movement opens your creativity, building self-confidence, and then self-respect always follows. Commit to daily movement: moving the body and coordinating your breathing with the movement. Consistent, daily practice opens the body to space. These sequences of movement will create openness for creativity and high performance throughout the day.

With these ritual the importance is not so much what you do, it's partaking of creative movement on a consistent basis. Daily consistent action 'maketh the man' – and the woman.

Daily Ritual 8: Body brushing

Cellular cleansing, detoxification through lymphasizing

The skin is the largest waste elimination organ in the body. The skin receives approximately a third of the blood circulated around the body. The skin is also the last organ to receive nutrients from the blood, but the first to show the lack of them. Think of the signs of aging: dry skin, irritated or itchy skin, in-growing hairs, and cellulite. Cellulite is a toxin accumulated in the body's fat cells. Brushing can help with tightening the skin, reducing the appearance of cellulite.

Daily brushing removes the dead skin that potentially clogs the pores and interfere with toxins being eliminated, so it can help the appearance and texture of the skin. Body brushing is therefore another way of detoxing your body and stimulating the lymphatic system. The lymphatic system transports immune cells throughout the body and supports the immune function.

Body brushing also aids muscle tone by distributing fat deposits more evenly across the body, and is a great rejuvenator of the nerve endings in the skin. It's especially beneficial for those who live a sedentary life. Little or no exercise and jobs that demand that you sit at a computer all day do no good for your posture.

ACTION

Buy an appropriate body brush (soft natural fibre, long-handled, removable head with strap).I have used many, but my favourite is a Japanese short-handled one.

Your skin must be dry, before your shower, bath or swim – this is easiest done naked.

Some research suggests circular movement, some suggests long sweeping strokes; some research suggests top to bottom, some suggests bottom to top; some research suggests starting with your extremities – your arms and legs, some suggests finishing there; some research suggest working left to right... Find what works for you, but always work towards the heart.

Please avoid sensitive areas such as sunburn, varicose veins, broken skin, inflamed skin, skin cancer, and genitalia.

Please also be careful and sensitive around the chest and breasts.

Some research suggests following up the brushing with bathing, a shower or a stint in the steam room, using hot and cold water to stimulate blood supply.

Some research advises moisturising your skin after your shower.

If you are feeling unwell, do this practice twice a day; it will boost the immune system, stimulating the body's natural healing process.

I adore this ritual. It is a daily must for me to body brush. It makes me feel alive within my body. The sensory feedback is wonderful. As I am brushing, I can feel the skin rejuvenating. Instant feedback. Be gentle, and love the skin you are in.

Daily Ritual 9: Purposeful beautiful breakfast

Breakfast is vital for creating an abundance of energy throughout the day. It is critical in sustaining healthy hormones and body chemicals. It is my favourite meal of the day. It fuels every cell in your body, preparing it for the extraordinary day ahead.

When clients come to me wanting to lose weight, this invariably will be an underlying factor: they do not eat breakfast.

On their first assessment, we discuss and document their activities of daily living.

To show the client what their food intake actually is, for a minimum of seven days they must keep a food diary. What we think we eat and what we really eat can sometimes be miles apart. Food diaries should record these details about what you have eaten:

1. Amount of food consumed
2. Your perception of your food
3. Eating breakfast regularly
4. Your feelings while preparing and eating
5. Length of time to eat your meals
6. When you ate
7. What time you woke up

8. How you felt when you woke
9. What time you went to bed
10. How you felt when going to bed

Many of my clients either do not have breakfast, or consume a huge quantity of empty calories within a small intake of food. A coffee shop latte and takeaway muffin are a perfect example of this: an immense number of calories with little or no nutritional gain.

I have been given every possible reason not to eat breakfast:

- I'm not a morning person.
- It makes me eat more during the day.
- It makes me go to the toilet when it's inconvenient to do so.
- It makes me want to poo, and I won't go anywhere else than at home.
- I don't have enough time in the mornings, what with getting kids ready and out of the house.
- I hate eating early in the mornings.
- I'm not hungry when I wake up.
- It makes me feel sick.
- Blah, blah blah...

Here are some symptoms clients reported when they haven't eaten breakfast:

- Pallor
- Agitation or anger
- Slight shakes and feeling irritable
- Lack of energy, weakness, fatigue, lethargy

- Slight confusion at times
- Lack of clarity of thought
- Low levels of concentration
- Excessive hunger

Skipping breakfast lowers certain chemicals in the brain that regulate food cravings and intake. You are guaranteed to eat more later in the day if you don't eat breakfast.

If you want to perform at your best throughout your day, eat breakfast. The ideal breakfast to have is one high in fat, with medium protein and low in carbohydrates. That means the cereals and fresh orange juice sold to us as healthy are definitely not. Eating traditional high-carbohydrate breakfast, such as 'healthy' cereals, milk, orange juice, encourages the body to store fat. These high levels of carbohydrate have an immediate effect on our fat-storing hormones. They also affect chemicals in our brain, creating feelings of sleepiness.

On the other hand, English breakfasts are a must.

A good breakfast is simple: create the environment to enjoy every moment of breakfast and eat the right things. No more cereals or orange juice.

Dairy (cheese, butter, cream, or full fat milk), meat, poultry, fish, eggs, served with vegetables cooked in coconut oil, will create optimum inner health. These foundational ingredients will take you on an exciting culinary journey heading towards optimum health. Your thoughts will be clearer, your energy levels abundant, and you will be fuelled to be your daily best.

Getting good fats into your body is vital to prime your body for peak performance through the day. This starts with the cooking oil: organic coconut oil is beautiful to cook with. It has a high burning rate and supports the body to release fat especially abdominal fat. Coconut oil has many known health benefits from reducing appetite to lowering cholesterol levels.

Birdonabike's Green Power Smoothie

Here is my Green Power Smoothie. I adore it. This is pure love being fed into my body every day.

(All the ingredients are organic):

- A blender: NutriBullet or similar
- 4-6 organic dates, stoned
- Juice of half a lemon (organic lemons will have more pips than others)
- A handful of spinach
- A handful of kale
- ½ cucumber
- ½ avocado(please take the skin off and the stone out)
- A handful of blanched almonds
- Fresh ginger to taste (I use an inch)
- A handful of fresh mint
- 4 ice cubes (I always filter my water)
- Water to taste (I love my smoothie thick enough to chew on)
- Ground flaxseed mix, any variety. This can be bought ready ground.

Blend everything together, except for the dates, adding more water to taste.

Add the dates after you have zapped all the ingredients together, and then blitz again in short, sharp bursts of power.

Sometimes I have this twice a day. You will feel every cell in your body go 'Aahhh, I am loved!'

Daily Ritual 10: Nutritional timing

Just like comedy, it's all about the timing.

Going to bed hungry

This is a ritual worthy of your commitment. You will wake up vibrating with energy. You will wake up excited to take on your best day. You will wake up with a morning song – come on, everyone has a morning song!

I know when I get my day aligned to my thoughts and actions, the knock-on effect on the following day is a guaranteed morning song. Every time! I have fallen in love with this ritual. Start your day with the question, 'What's my morning song?' You will be surprised. You've just got to listen.

It can be painful to start with. We modern humans dislike being hungry. The first three days of practicing this ritual are super-challenging, but the rewards awaiting you are truly amazing. You will come to enjoy the sense of lightness, of space and of feeling free within.

Allowing the body to rest its digestive system is vital for hormone manipulation. The body releases a hormone required for cellular repair, controlling your metabolism and growth: growth hormone. Growth hormone enhances and stimulates the way fat is used within the body.

During the first part of your sleep, growth hormone is at its highest levels. That's why it is super-important not to eat too close to bedtime. To take this further, avoid caffeine or alcohol in the three hours before you go to bed. Research shows not consuming caffeine and alcohol for four to six hours before bedtime leads to optimum health, fat loss and an energy boost. To get the best out of this process, create a regular sleeping and waking pattern.

This ritual is an absolute must for optimum health. Being at your peak of fitness requires your body to be clean and lean. Think of your body as trillions of cells, not as a single entity. It is your duty to keep every cell clean and lean to fulfill your dreams, creating energy like you have never felt before.

Optimum health and peak performance come from keeping the cells clean and nourished at all times. You should be detoxing your cells every day.

What you do every day creates the body you find yourself in?

Daily Ritual 11: Being mindful

Daily reflection

The night is closing in. It's a great time to sit in a quiet, peaceful spot in your home.

If it's like my household, it is busy, noisy, with guitars jamming, conversation/shouting from room to room, a hairdryer blowing, people hollering 'Mum!', and aliens, sorry, children, invading every inch of the house...

Go and create a space, even if it is your bed – just somewhere you can go to where your mind and body know that this is time for peace. Many think you should not make your bed your space of peace. You make your space of peace wherever you want to – if your bed is the only plot of land in your house to call your own, grab it with both hands.

Now you have created 'your space', personalize it. Own your peace space. I have created a small shrine to the devotion of *Me*. Well, that's not strictly true, but I have placed candles, personalized crystals and my daily books on a tall, narrow bedroom cabinet. I have a love affair with books, and with my cat. I know, 'Get a life!'

I adore two books written by women for daily use throughout the year:

Julia Cameron's *The Artist's Way Every Day: A year of creative living*

Sarah Ban Breathnach's *Simple Abundance: A daybook of comfort and joy*

I read them both as I am setting up to write in the mornings and, keeping in the flow of this daily ritual, read them during my reflection time at night. Sometimes I read them both morning and night.

I urge you to seek out yearly daybooks that stir your emotions, that you can connect with, that sweep away any feelings of isolation by showing you you are not the only person on the planet.

Once you have set up 'your peace space' and you've personalized it with creative objects, books, trinkets and candles, find yourself a blanket or a pashmina/throw. You must be warm. It's always a challenge for me to be warm. I hope you can visualize me, sitting upright on my bed in a lilac pashmina, with my candles and crystals, and not forgetting Chicken (the cat, of course) snuggled on my lap.

Now you are ready to begin reflecting on the day that was.

Daily reflection allows you to keep your focus on your goals. During this time of reflection, you breathe and allow your memories to flow. Distractions occur throughout our busy lives. We are busy being busy and our focus is taken away from our vision of our dreams. Documenting your thoughts, feelings, dreams and passions helps your practice of daily reflection, giving you a reference point. When you fall off the pathway to your purpose, which will happen, you can be guided back on to it.

ACTION

Conscious breathing

This takes 5 minutes. Sit in your reflection area/peace space, drawing your attention to your breathing: how the breath flows into the body and then is released.

Become aware of the depth of your breath. Close your eyes as you breathe.

Set 2 minutes on your alarm for this exercise. If you are finding 2 minutes too long, do not resist. Do 1 minute, building up over the first week. Soon, 1 minute will not be enough.

Sit in peace, palms facing up to the universe, breathing and reflecting for 2 minutes. Enjoy.

Practise breathing first, then reflection and writing in your diary, or vice-versa. This is something you must play with and decide what is right for you. You may find that the evening is not the right time for you. Mornings before the rest of the house wakes can peaceful. These suggestions are here to support you to develop your own personal daily rituals. All of these rituals are for you to call your own, for you to put into practice and make a considered decision on whether they contribute to your goals.

Gratitude diary

Is there a difference between a gratitude diary and a journal? Surely it's the same process. In a word, no. They are completely different.

A gratitude diary is a great source of inspiration, encouraging you to focus on the positive l areas in your life, whether it's the simple things or more significant aspects.

'Give thanks for a little, and you will find a lot.'

Hausa proverb

There are many ways to keep a gratitude journal. It is not a reflective diary, or a diary of your activities during the day. It's a way of being thankful, of providing a personal focus for gratitude.

Robert Emmons, one of the leading experts on the science of gratitude, has documented all the top research-based tips for reaping psychological rewards from keeping a gratitude journal. He has developed a 21-day programme for creating emotional prosperity through recording gratitude.

Here are some keys points, in no particular order, for keeping a gratitude diary:

1. Be consistent, writing in your journal every day, preferably at the same time of day, preferably in the evening (although some research has shown that you only need to write in your journal twice a week. It's your choice).
2. Don't just go through the motions: making a decision to become happier helps with this exercise.
3. Focus on people rather than things.
4. Focus on your surroundings.
5. Some researchers say to keep it simple and list no more than five things, others say there should be no limits. Some days will be full, others not so much.
6. Be creative: use surprises. This creates a stronger response.
7. Don't see it as a chore – vary the sorts of things you include.
8. Turn negatives into positives.

I always start my gratitude diary with: 'Today I am most thankful for... '

Even when you are feeling that you have just had the worst of days, or you are so exhausted that even keeping your eyes open is pain, write your gratitude diary.

As with all of the daily rituals, start small, allow yourself to achieve them, and the magic will happen.

Bird's 'had enough' moment

I started this ritual three years ago. I had heard and read about amazing changes to people's lives from keeping a gratitude diary, from attitudes changing, a change in business success, to communicating with your loved ones more effectively.

I started writing lists, numbering each thought, but not elaborating or going into detail. This soon evolved into a deeper, more meaningful description of events or observations that I encountered during my day. I found focusing on writing a short list gave me the skill to identify what I was actually grateful for. I researched at length how to do it, why, when, and what to include. In the end, it came down to just doing it. Many people think you should not repeat the same thoughts, but this created a problem for me. It made the whole process stilted. It stopped my writing flowing. I removed this barrier and just wrote whatever thoughts flowed.

Countless times at the beginning I couldn't see what I had to be grateful for. At this time in my life, the children and I had to leave the family home because of a damaging marriage. My husband had refused to leave. I had no family living locally to support me, nowhere to go quickly, and I was keen not to cause too much disruption to the children. I was worried about how this would affect Jack, as he had been admitted to a psychiatric hospital the year before. I was in terrible emotional pain, leaving a man I loved, but circumstances had forced my hand. I had little money, certainly no deposit for emergency accommodation, and minimal furniture.

I'm sure you would agree that coming up with feelings of gratitude at this period was a tall order.

In desperation, willing to try anything and everything to stop the pain, I started the diary: a list of short and succinct observations, with very little emotion.

The power of observation

Here's the big but. I wrote about how grateful I was to have supportive friends, extraordinary children, love, understanding and generous clients, and my personal hope began to grow.

On some days, when it all got too much, I was thankful for the most basic of human needs: life, oxygen and the ability to breathe. Some days that's all I felt I could do: breathe. I wrote it down: breathing. No more needed to be said.

I started to look around. I found the simplest of gestures from people created momentum to carry me through the day. They inspired in me an abundance of gratitude, and gratitude leads to hope.

I drew on external sources of gratitude: the beautiful town we lived in, the weather, the wonderful rolling hills, and the dramatic coastline that surrounded me.

This shift in focus made a big impact on my state. Tony Robbins often talks about your state and the speed with which you can change it. Your state dictates your day. Your state dictates the decisions you make. Your state alters your perception.

After a week of writing lists in my gratitude diary, I began to expand on my day. It became quite in-depth, with 'he said', and 'she said'; it was evolving into an autobiography of gratitude. It seemed my change of state and focus changed the world around me. Great opportunities arose; joy and peace filled my soul. I valued this daily ritual so highly, I took my diary on holiday. Regardless of how tired I was of an evening, my commitment to being grateful was relentless.

This all came crashing down when I had a shoulder operation and was immobile, doubled up with excruciating pain. My gratitude diary became a daily ritual I failed to practise. My habit of writing late into the evening became a despised activity. I no more wanted to spend time with my thoughts – making up how wonderful things were and saying how blessed I was – than I wanted to eat my own young.

In the end, I got sick of feeling this way. I had evidence of the great results from recording gratitude. I knew you couldn't attract the things you don't have. I could see before me the need, at these darkest of times, to focus on the good. I took the practice of writing a gratitude journal back to its basics. I began writing, in list format, five things/thoughts that I was grateful for, rather than recording my daily activities. This was about noting down my feelings. I was totally aware of my resistance to this practice. I acknowledged my feelings, making sure not to dismiss them. I knew I must break through this mini failure, as enlightenment was waiting.

ACTION

Making a gratitude list

Take 2 minutes, following your 2-minute evening reflection, to

sit peacefully in the late evening, smile, and begin to list five thoughts, things, people, or events that that you encountered during your day. Make the list short and to the point, with minimal detail.

To progress this practice, list as many things as you like.

To progress it further, develop your list into one-page journal inserts, detailing your feelings and thoughts, and how these will shape your future.

Prepare for tomorrow today

Preparing should be your last ritual of the day.
Preparing your thoughts of tomorrow today.
Preparing your body's nervous system for tomorrow.
Preparing your energy for tomorrow.
Write with a pen and notebook, not on electronic devices.

Research shows that writing with a pen and paper is more beneficial to our focus and memory. Writing stimulates the area at the base of our brain, known as the reticular activating system, which is a filter for all the information the brain needs to process. This brings focus to our work and enhances memory.

ACTION

Preparing for tomorrow

Choose a beautiful journal or notebook. The colour of paper adds to the creativity of this activity.(Many artists write on yellow paper.)

Use your diary, and transfer your day tomorrow, the night before. This primes and engages your focus on the day ahead. Keeping you aligned with your vision.

Take no more than 5 minutes to prepare for tomorrow, today.

Enjoy every moment.

If you want to bounce out of bed, excited with clarity for the day ahead, make this daily ritual a must.

* * *

These 11 daily rituals, practised every day, will create a body that is clean, lean and has an abundance of energy such as you have never felt before.

This is pure optimum health.

Book trail

Banting, W. and Meadows, W. (2015). *The Banting Diet: Letter on corpulence.* CreateSpace Independent Publishing Platform. (Kindle edition available)

Hamilton, D. R. (2008). *How Your Mind Can Heal Your Body.* London: Hay House. (Kindle edition available)

Hay, L. (2013). *Heal Your Body.* London: Hay House. (Kindle edition available)

Kelder, P. (2011). *Ancient Secret of the Fountain of Youth. London: Virgin Books.* (Kindle edition available)

Kelder, P. (2008). The Eye of Revelation: The ancient Tibetan rites of rejuvenation. Bradenton, FL: Booklocker. (Kindle edition available) Reprinted from the expanded 1946 edition

Kilham, C.S. (2011). *The Five Tibetans: Five dynamic exercises for health, energy and personal power.* Rochester: Healing Arts Press. (Kindle edition available)

Levy, T.E. (2011*). Curing the Incurable: Vitamin C, infectious diseases and toxins.* Henderson, NV: MedFox Publishing.

Yan Ming, S. S., (2006). The Shaolin Workout: 28 days to transforming your body, mind and spirit with kung-fu. Emmaus, PA: Rodale. (Kindle edition available)

10

I Know You Know I Know You Know

Look inside yourself, Simba, you are more than what you have become.'

Mufasa, *The Lion King*

Human beings are social animals. You are not an island.

According to Aristotle, 'Man is by nature a social animal; an individual who is unsocial naturally and not accidentally is either beneath our notice or more than human. Society is something that precedes the individual. Anyone who either cannot lead the common life or is so self-sufficient as not to need to, and therefore does not partake of society, is either a beast or a god.'

We find ourselves in relationships within our environment on a daily basis. In the Daily Rituals, your environment was your body, your internal environment. Now you will see how you can affect your internal environment by how you choose to behave in your external environment. You can influence and adapt your external environment. You are a super-powerful being. Your behaviour can achieve what you choose to believe.

The way we use body language can create an internal energy. Adapting your body language to how you want to feel on a daily basis has a nuclear impact on your thoughts, feelings and actions. Maybe you question these words. 'Surely your thoughts create your actions?' I hear you say – and you would be correct. To adapt your body language is reverse engineering: another tool to create your desired feelings.

Our wellbeing depends on the quality of our relationships, from our intimate relationships to our exchange with the shop assistant. It is imperative for us to form connections with others. Connecting, touching, meeting with others generates a surge of energy through you.

Robert Waldinger, in his recent TED talk, unveiled findings from the longest longitudinal study on adult development. The study is continuing into its 75th year, following a number of men throughout their lives. It has demonstrated that good relationships keep us happier and healthier. But the study went deeper into the findings to uncover three main lessons:

Lesson 1: Social relationships are good for our happiness and health

Community has a positive influence on our physical health, helping us to live longer and happier lives. Loneliness kills. Loneliness is toxic. It has a direct effect on the decline of our health and brain function, leading to shorter lives. In the USA one in five people report being lonely.

Lesson 2: Quality of relationships

It is not how many friends you have but the quality of the relationships that matters. Living in conflict in a marriage can be more detrimental to health than divorce.

Lesson 3: The men most satisfied in their relationships at the age of 50 were the healthiest at the age of 80.

Could it be that quality relationships are anti-ageing? Build quality relationships within your environment and health and happiness will follow.

I love connecting with everyone I meet in my day. Saying 'hello' is such a kind gift to share with a passer-by. Talking to the checkout lady is energizing. Forming informal connections with strangers is empowering. It makes you feel amazing. The energy you give and receive from forming kind connections is visible. The charge you get from other humans and animals is overwhelming. Throughout our bodies, each cell creates vibrations of energy. When we connect, forming a relationship with other living beings, the charge can be given and received with great force. There are certain people you meet with whom the exchange of energy is on the scale of a nuclear reaction. Purely by forming connections with others, our own personal energy levels are elevated to wondrous heights.

Personal energy freemiums

I was brought up in the West Country (Devon and Cornwall), where everybody greets you with 'Hello, my luvver' – a warm, welcoming, feel-good greeting – and asks about your day. I lived in a small town where everybody knew everybody knew everybody. The pace of life was slow and walking with ease was a must. Popping into a friend's house for a cup of tea uninvited is welcomed as a thoughtful gesture. My granddad always said he would do things 'directly' (said in a Cornish accent and pronounced 'dre-ckly'). This actually means it will never get done, but the love and care are there.

I continued to use this kindness wherever the wind took me. On moving to Kent, the Garden of England, I found these friendly gestures to be alien to the locals, even in a small-town environment. It seems the busy, fast pace; the rude, intrinsic lonely London feel, have spilled over to its surrounding towns. Apparently you don't speak to people you don't know, especially if you're on the London Underground. People look at you as if you have two heads – and that's just if you smile at someone. I found this affected my emotions; I felt crushed and it actually affected my energy.

I made a conscious decision to continue to show respect and love for all the connections I made and for my established relationships. This is part of my daily practice: giving respect and love to other human beings, no matter who they are or how they feel about me or behave towards me.

Oprah Winfrey, in her wonderful book *What I Know For Sure* says she is

'willing to see the best in people, regardless of them showing their worst'. Breathe those words in. Let them wash over you and take root in your thoughts. These words make me tingle – I have made them my own: 'Always see the best even when being shown the worst'.

Being aware of my feelings and how they affect my thoughts and actions has supported me in forming and maintaining daily friendly relationships.

ACTION

Write down in your journal your thoughts and feelings about forming relationships with other human beings, no matter who they are, from the local grocery shop assistant to your company director.

- How do you behave?
- How do you communicate?
- How does that make you feel?
- How would you like to feel?
- How would you like to leave that person feeling?

'Smile and Wave, Boys, Smile and Wave'

Madagascar

It's super-simple. Practise this with each person that you pass throughout your day. It's so energizing to you and to the person you're greeting.

- Adopt great posture: body upright, head up.
- Look at the other person and keep eye contact for two to four seconds.
- Smile (try not to wave).
- Greet them with a warm 'hello'.
- Wait for it to land on them.

Prepare for the surprised reaction from them. You will either receive a return greeting, or you clearly are not speaking English and you will – wait for it – be ignored.

I prefer receiving a greeting rather than being blanked. But really I just love to give; in fact when I am not consistent in this behaviour I experience unease. It's a must for me to form a connection with all the people that I have contact with in my day. It brings me great joy, and joy is a core desired feeling for me.

This practice of greeting strangers can become addictive. My clients laugh so much when we are out training together: will they or won't they reply?

The wonderful energy generated by this practice creates a ripple effect in your community. Wait till popping into your friends for a cuppa uninvited becomes more widespread and accepted. It will go viral!

The look

Eye contact is the most powerful of non-verbal communication. Ralph Waldo Emerson wrote 'The eyes of men converse as much as their tongues.' Eye contact gives you an immediate connection with another human. To develop your practice in eye contact, connect your glance with another's for a minimum of 8, but no more than 10 seconds. This skill is super-powerful but when you are starting out it can make you feel uncomfortable; 8-10 seconds are like an eternity. Start small (2 seconds at a time) and build from there.

ACTION

Take 2 minutes

Choose your target wisely: it should be someone you are familiar with. Build slowly, starting as suggested with 2–5 seconds. I guarantee you will laugh within an instant.

Ask for feedback from your target and consider your own reaction. Record and compare your findings as you develop the practice.

Those you surround yourself with, you become

I'm sure you have heard that you become the sum of the five people closest to you. It's even suggested that your income is the mean of that of your five closest friends. It's such an interesting concept, and one that I have been developing for some time.

On first coming into contact with this concept, I felt unease and resistance inside. Tony Robbins introduced it to me at my first 'Unleash the Power Within' event. Within the first four hours of the event, attendees are primed and inspired to walk over burning coals, as a metaphor that everything is possible. While networking at the event I came across many experienced 'Firewalkers' who shared with me the piece of wisdom that had had the biggest impact on them. 'Go and surround yourself with higher beings,' they said – those with more success, more passion, more wealth, greater physical health and fitness, better quality relationships and more fulfilment in their lives. This made me protective of the friends

I already had. I felt huge intrinsic resistance. I even questioned my integrity at this potentially dismissive attitude towards my current relationships. But with unwavering faith in my values and beliefs, I gently introduced this concept, all the while being kind to myself and staying in alignment with who I am.

Now I rejoice in this process. I see the value in surrounding yourself with people who are more advanced in the areas of your life that you wish to develop. It can still at times make me feel nervous or self-doubting, but I have come to be addicted to these contacts. The energy they bring will generate greatness. My nan always said, 'Great oaks from little acorns grow'.

ACTION

Breathe. Become aware of the breath in your body and how it makes you feel.

Then take 2 minutes to ask yourself the following questions:

- Who do I spend most time with in my day?
- Breathe and release
- Who do I surround myself with?
- Breathe
- What are the qualities of the relationships?
- Breathe
- Are my friendships quality connections?
- Breathe
- What are my values and beliefs for friendships?

- Breathe
- What are my expectations of my friendships?
- Breathe

Write your answers in your journal and date them.
Please revisit what you have written. Be sure to note down the date of each occasion that you do so. These will be nuggets of gold for you. Otherwise, I promise you, you will forget the feelings you had at any given moment.

To thine own self be true

This was truly challenging for me, especially after my divorce. Many of my dearest friends were busy in their own lives. I was no longer able to sustain our friendship: no more dinner parties, no more couple suppers out. I found myself trying to give, but I was not offering what they wanted to receive so I distanced myself, making myself into an island for my own protection. I was fearful of more rejection. Of course, my fears became reality, with unbearable pain in tow.

I often reassess this tricky time in my life. I valued and adored my friendships – they were like a comfortable hot water bottle. My perception of giving was not what my friends perceived. Who I am as a person became lost in translation; my friends became blind to me. Later I came to understand that I was not fulfilling my friends' needs for certainty and connection. My rapid transformation was alien to them, something they were unable to process. By disconnecting myself for self-preservation, I created unease and a sense of rejection for my friends. They were amazingly kind people, with the best of intentions, yet they could not see past my self-isolation to my goodness.

I was able to understand this challenging discomfort, but I found it painful most of the time. Then came clarity and after that an understanding of myself. I could witness and feel their pain too. I even understood it. I loved my friends, but they were too close to me see me clearly, so with kindness and love I gave them permission to leave me, so that the future would lead us to recovery.

Have you got friends that do not see you, but come to your relationship with kindness and good intentions? Are you meeting their needs? What are their needs?

No need to reply – just pursue your dialogue internally. As Ramadas sang on one of the most life-transforming documentaries I have ever seen, 'What about me, what about me, what about me?' In 2002 Jamie Catto released a film, *One Giant Leap*, accompanied by the most touching music, depicting the complexities of humans and the connections they form. I share this with you as it was shared with me, with love and grace: you must watch this film.

Maslow's Hierarchy of Needs, articulated in 1954, suggests that if our basic need for connection is not met, we are unable to focus on progressing to the higher levels of motivation and the pursuit of betterment. Max Neef has developed further the psychology of human needs. He classifies the fundamental human needs as:

- Subsistence
- Protection

- Affection
- Understanding
- Participation
- Leisure
- Creation
- Identity
- Freedom

There could be a complete mismatch between your needs and those of your friend, leading each of you to be unable to comprehend the other.

ACTION

Take 5 minutes to consider the fundamentals of human need and ask yourself if you are fulfilling the needs of your close relationships. 'Making sense', Jonathan Haidt calls it. Make sense of your relationships. Understand and build on the areas of need. Write your thoughts in your journal and date them.

Masterminding

Masterminding is not a quiz for highly intellectual individuals! Masterminding is 'a composite mind, consisting of two or more individuals working in perfect harmony with a definite aim in view'. It is obvious that bringing a group of minds together will create an abundance of power. Napoleon Hill perceived that great power can only be accumulated through this principle. Proximity is power.

Napoleon Hill showed the value of masterminding and how success follows from using the 'Driving Force'. It was the ninth step towards riches in his book *Think And Grow Rich* and features in *The Magic Ladder To Success.* In this he categorizes Masterminding as his first lesson in the Law of Success.

It is on record that Henry Ford and Thomas Edison were personal friends who created their own personal 'Mastermind' between them. This grew to involve Harvey Firestone, Luther Burbank and John Burroughs, each contributing their great brainpower.

Although there are many claims as to who was in the first reported Mastermind group, Benjamin Franklin in the early 1700s seems to have the edge. His collaboration did not did not go by the name 'Masterminding'; it was called the Leather Apron Club, and evolved into Junto. Personally, I believe King Arthur and The Round Table beat them all to it!

A Masterminding group is formed when everyone comes together to give and to serve the group in a focused way. Each individual is given a time allocation in which they can share a thought or question that the group then reflects on, offering guidance, advice and support. There are conditions for the topic: it could be business related, personal or social. The practice gives scope for the free share of information.

Joint ventures are planned; friendships are formed, allowing ideas to float freely without the worry of stealing intellectual property. Rapport is developed within the group. Henry Ford said, 'Coming together is a beginning, keeping together is progress, working together is success.' Masterminding allows you to surround yourself with a higher-level playing field.

It sounds so easy – just go and get some people who are more successful in life than you and make a group! It is challenging, at first, to find the right people, and then to form a group. I started off in a large group and elevated myself within this group of entrepreneurs. I invested my money and, more importantly, my time in finding extraordinary people. It felt truly uncomfortable, but this is where I knew growth would come from.

This has been one of the most challenging shifts in my personal transformation. I felt guilty about wanting to be around people more successful in business or wealth. But to be surrounded by extraordinary human beings striving for levels of excellence; to share ideas, knowledge, ideologies, and to wrap yourself in their cloak of energy – this search for excellence became a source of immense power.

I still valued my friends, but to take myself to the next level of my life I had to come out of my comfort zone. Placing myself in the transformation zone of raised questions such as, 'What can I bring to these (in my opinion) highly successful people? What knowledge can I share?'

In this state of confusion, uncomfortable thoughts can be exciting. Prepare for your energy to explode during the process of personal growth.

The wonderful joy a Mastermind group brings comes from its egalitarian approach. All the ideas shared are worthy of consideration and no one sits in judgment. The purpose of the group is for ideas to be given life and energy, filling the air with creative thinking.

With unwavering faith, go and immerse yourself in an environment that will inspire you to succeed. As a leader, a visionary, go and bring your magnificent dreams to life.

Book trail

Benner, J. (2015). *The Impersonal Life.* New York: Merchant Books. (Kindle edition available) This book was originally published anonymously in 1941 but after his death the author's wife revealed his name.

Dyer, W.W. (2009). *Your Erroneous Zones: Escape negative thinking and take control of your life.* London: Piatkus Books. (Kindle edition available)

Foundation for Inner Peace (1992). *A Course in Miracles* (combined volume). London: Arkana.

Gladwell, M. (2002). *The Tipping Point: How little things can make a big difference.* New York: Abacus Books. (Kindle edition available)

Henry, T. (2015). *Die Empty: Unleash your best work every day.* New York: Portfolio. (Kindle edition available)

Henry, T. (2015). *Louder than Words: Harness the power of your authentic voice.* New York: Portfolio. (Kindle edition available)

Hill, N. (2007). *Think and Grow Rich.* Radford, VA: Wilder Publications. (Kindle edition available) Originally published in 1937.

Moorjani, A. (2012). *Dying To Be Me: My journey from cancer, to near death, to true healing.* London: Hay House. (Kindle edition available)

Nepo, M. (2000). *The Book of Awakening: Having the life you want by being present in the life you have.* Berkeley, CA: Conari Press. (Kindle edition available)

Sharma, R. (2015). *The Monk Who Sold His Ferrari.* London: Harper Thorsons. (Kindle edition available)

The Master Number

'Remember, you're the one who can fill the world with sunshine.'

Snow White

Numerology is the science behind numbers and letters that can unleash the potential in your life.

The final chapter, finishing on a number 11, uses the power of numerology to support you on your onward journey.

This 'master' number in numerology makes double use of the number one, which means new beginnings and is considered the most intuitive number of all numbers. It represents a balance of energy internally and in your surrounding environment. The number is associated with faith, instinct, charisma and dynamism.

What I know to be real are the little incremental gains, the simple support from external factors, that make immeasurable contributions to your progress.

Using the number 11 to inspire you to begin, to take action, to choose, will create so much energy to help you become your daily best.

Who makes you smile?

Who do you love?
Who do you aspire to be?
Who is aligned with you and your values?
Whose words reach into your soul and grab your heart?
Who makes you smile?
Who makes you say, 'I want to be like you when I grow up'?

I adore, read and listen to Coco Chanel, Audrey Hepburn, Marie Forleo, Liz DiAlto, Oprah Winfrey and Sarah Ban Breathnach. But I wake to the wondrous words of my hero, Benjamin Franklin: 'What good shall I do this day?' This is my waking thought, the words that greet me on my walls.

ACTION

Take 5 minutes to write the answers to these questions in your journal:

- Who is your hero?
- Who do you aspire to be?
- Who would you model to grow into yourself?

Sir Richard Branson is the face of a brand that I associate with fun. What a wonderful business philosophy to be aligned with! In an interview on success, he gave three achievable outcomes that anyone could aspire to in their business.

1. Understand your calculated risks. Can you survive the downside of your business?
2. Be the best in everything you do.
3. Really make a difference.

His words excite me. His words make everything possible. His words make me smile.

Becoming a Magic Memory Maker

You are a hero to those around you. You achieve more than any other person you know. You have the ability to make conscious decisions. You are a super-successful woman, reaching heights most cannot even see. Now prepare to become the superhero, Magic Moment Maker. Your family will love this concept.

My little people always remember the magic moments – not the many presents that cost a fortune, but the funny times spent together.

Giving your time, being present in your family is the greatest gift – I mean really present, not just there in body. Being present, engaging, listening, smiling, laughing and giving all those wonderful special hugs. This doesn't mean being there in person, but taking your mobile office with you. This means not checking emails, not answering mobile calls from clients or finding reasons why you have to work. I accept that there always are reasons, but just being there will not make you into the Magic Moment Maker.

I have so many magic moments to share. Of course going to Disney World in Florida is creating magic moments through spending huge amounts of money, but a professional Magic Moment Maker needs more than the expensive holiday to create those smiles that make you glow inside. Money couldn't buy any of my most treasured memories.

My granddad could make a whistle from a birch tree branch. I mean, it could make music; it was truly a work of art.

ACTION

Take 5 minutes to record your thoughts on becoming a Magic Memory Maker:

- What would your family love to do with you?
- What would you love to do with your family?
- How can you record the moments?
- How can you make your family smile, and give a proper belly laugh?

We all love going to the cinema. Our car journey home is always a passionate discussion about which bit was our magic moment in the film. We spend the whole car journey home in a heated debate, with everybody getting a chance to air their views.

You can develop this skill of creating magic moments from your day. It's a powerful way of debriefing from your day. It's very similar to your gratitude diary, a way of acknowledging the wonder of your day.

Be true to yourself

But who are you?

Have you heard of the 'I am' story? 'I am... ?'

It's a powerful, fundamental question. And this is an extraordinary exercise of self-discovery, one that is a must to record and revisit. This quest, this question, goes with you through your life. It is how you identify yourself.

How do you know if you are being true to yourself if you have not identified what that looks like to you? Identify yourself to you. You are what you identify with, staying consistent with your self-identity.

Be clear on seeing things for what they are. Tell yourself the truth. To discover who you really are is liberating. To know your-self is to be your-self. All of this sounds so easy, but to go there and find the strength to discover yourself can be exhausting and scary.

What if you find someone you do not recognize or, worse, don't like?

Victoria's 'had enough' moment

Victoria's worth was invested in her job title. She was super successful in a male-dominated workplace and very proud to be the equal of her husband in terms of salary. A mother of three, she would return home super-fatigued after 10 hours at work. She drank a bottle of wine a night to de-stress, and was unable to switch off until just after midnight.

Suffering chronic back problems, she was unable to sustain movement for longer than 20 minutes and heavily overweight. She was totally disgusted by her body, and did not feel womanly either in herself or in relation to her partner. Needless to say, her relationship was compromised in some areas. Nevertheless, feeding her family organic produce was a must for her, although when time was not on her side, she had to settle for less.

I started addressing Victoria's limited mobility. She was unable to walk with her family, or take the dog for a walk. Her pain was unbearable most days, and only manageable at all thanks to quarterly injections. Surgery was an option offered to this relatively young woman, but fear that it would not be a complete success made her turn down the specialists.

I started her on daily gentle movement, alongside a training plan for achieving Victoria's outcomes. Interestingly, her weight, although it affected her appearance and her self-esteem, was something Victoria was not prepared to tackle.

Then, as so often, the universe took charge. It was not that Victoria listened to her body; it wasn't the pain stimulus, the weight stimulus, or the sadness that tipped the balance. Her role as a business woman was suddenly swept away from under her feet. Redundancy loomed, and with it the loss of identity, worth, value, equality.

What a wonderful gift to be given!

Now Victoria could begin to listen to her body; firstly, to understand that value does not come from what you are, but what you believe inside. Victoria needed to think, feel and believe that she was amazing, regardless of the external factors. This was the beginning of Victoria becoming her daily best.

Who we believe ourselves to be controls our lives; it guides our thoughts and feelings. You live by what you choose to believe. Do you identify with your job, your relationships? Keep a watch on how this develops.

Knowing who you are, your thoughts and feelings, your values and beliefs, guides you to pure energy, to finding your passion.

To have a passion is a gift, to yourself and to your environment. It doesn't just find you one day. You have to build emotional fitness, build emotional muscle day by day.

You must have absolute faith in the process of being your own personal gym. Your truth lies within you. You must visit your inner thoughts, to build your emotional and spiritual muscle. This is no different from any other muscle-building exercise. You must challenge the muscle consistently, adapting the daily exercises and allowing your thoughts to rest and recover. Pure emotional muscle power requires nurturing, love and patience. It has taken you years to store your emotions so beautifully deep within; it's going to take time to discover and understand them.

This is finding true courage. Remember, the word 'courage' comes from the Old French, meaning 'from the heart'.

Of my women clients, 80% come to me for quick and easy strategies for weight loss. But it's never about the weight loss; it's about the feelings they experience when they achieve the end results.

When I ask about their weight history, do I find that it has gone on quickly? Of course not: it has been a gradual process. Yet some women's perception of time becomes the source of their failure. They only start to pay attention of to themselves when they reach the point of desperation, and an inability to cope with themselves and the way they feel; or when they have reached their 'had enough' moment. Weight very rarely goes on quickly. It is a slow, incremental process. Some research shows the human body stores 2lbs of fat a year. Dr Stephen Guyenet suggests that the fat increase spikes during the holiday season. He states that 'most people don't put weight on overnight, it happens over years and decades.' We want instant results but the reality of the weight loss process is as slow and steady as that for gaining weight.

This goes against everything these women want. I call it the 'McDonald's effect':

1. Time is a factor.
2. The cost is a factor
3. The level of service is a factor
4. The result is a factor.
5. The feelings you experience are a factor.

McDonald's are wonderful at remembering what it is you are buying. You are buying time. What they provide is quick; it fulfills your need to feel full rather than hungry.

But it does not bring you the feelings you want to feel about yourself. It will not bring you the energy you want to feel on a daily basis. It will not bring you the health you aspire to for yourself and your family. The McDonald's effect stands in the way of your end result.

ACTION

This is where you will grow.

Use the 3Bs in the peaceful space within your home. Write your responses in your journal and put a date on your journal entries. I promise you, you will return to them at some point in wonder,

– Breathe.
Who am I?
– Breathe.
I am...
– Breathe.

As my training buddies say on race day, 'Leave it all out there.'

This action creates similar feelings to tidying up a messy room. The process starts with excitement. You can visualize the end result and you launch yourself in with vigour. Half way through, you're in detest mode; you're angry, so angry you are super-emotional, close to tears. Others may want your input, but your patience is at an all-time low. You carry on. You feel you have limited choice in the matter. With renewed effort, momentum gathers and the room begins to clear. The end is in sight (insight?); you begin to see before you. Clarity gives you power.

You feel amazing, energetic... and you have created space.

What Do I Do Now?

That's up to you. Your choice!

I have shared wisdom from my experiences with the most magnificent people and from the scholars that I have read. You now have the power of choice.

- Which daily ritual to incorporate into your day?
- Which exercise to practise first?
- Which quote burrows deep into your soul?
- When to practise?
- When to share the wisdom?
- Who to share it with?

Of all the words I have shared with you, the word 'choice' is the most prescriptive one. Choice gives you the power of making a decision. There is nothing worse than the pain of indecisiveness.

'The risk of a wrong decision is preferable to the terror of indecision.'

Maimonides (Spanish philosopher, 1204)

This I know to be true: pain cannot exist where unwavering faith and focus are present. You have followed your heart throughout these pages.

You have practised and set yourself apart each time you did so. You have explored and discovered your thoughts, your feelings, and your playful side. You have found an inner strength you never suspected in yourself before. You have listened to your words and created daily strategies.

Now what do you do?

- You begin from the essence of the breath.
- You listen to your body.
- You kill with kindness.

It always comes down to today, this moment.

- What you choose to think.
- What you choose to feel.
- What you choose to do.

These three elements of your life create an abundance of energy, create a love like nothing you have ever felt, so that you become your children's inspiration.

Go shine your light bright.

Book trail

Coyle, D. (2010). *The Talent Code: Greatness isn't born; it's grown.* London: Arrow Books. (Kindle edition available)

Frankl, V. E. (2004). *Man's Search for Meaning.* London: Rider Books. (Kindle edition available)

Gerber, M. E. (1988). *The E-Myth: Why most businesses don't work and what to do about it.* London: Harper Business.

Lao Tzu (1993). *Tao Te Ching.* Indianapolis: Hackett Publishing. (Kindle edition available)

Pressfield, S. (2012). *The War of Art: Break through the blocks and win your inner creative battles.* Black Irish Entertainment LLC. (Kindle edition available)

Pressfield, S. (2012). *Turning Pro: Tap you inner power and create your life's work.* Black Irish Entertainment LLC. (Kindle edition available)

Smart, J. (2013). *Clarity: Clear mind, better performance, bigger results.* Chichester: Capstone Publishing. (Kindle edition available)

Acknowledgements

I am truly blessed to be able to say thank you.

I have loved every moment of this process. From writing 1000 words a day for 30 days, to re-writing it all over again.

So here goes with my whole heart, to my children Jack, Olivia and Louis, hear these words: **you are so loved**.

To my best friend, Andrew David Young. Always baby. I can't wait to see your book on the big screen.

To my mother who has shown me eloquence of words, although I may not have always actioned your beautiful tone.

To Chicken, my gift of love all bundled up on four hairy legs. I adore meditating with you every morning.

To my friends, from the funny stories of snowboarding to dancing on the fridge. I appreciate your wonder and making magic moments.

To Entrevo and KPI, Daniel Priestley, Marcus Ubl, Darshana Ubl, Andrew Priestley and fellow entrepreneurs, you have given your wisdom with love and made me dig deep into the gold of business.

To Sammie, your amazing creations have brought to life these pages.

To the magnificent women who have shared their souls to me. I saw in you what you couldn't see. I knew what you did not know. I had faith where you had none. **You are enough**.

The Author

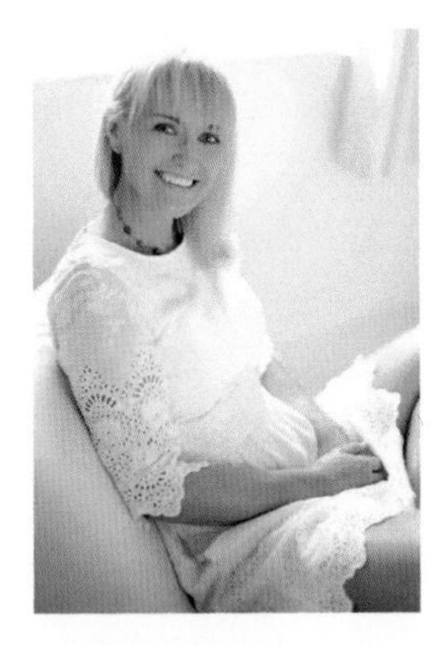

From the age of 14, Sarah-Anne Lucas wanted to be a nurse. Watching a TV programme called *Angels*, she thought they looked beautiful in their caps and capes. She graduated in 1995, only to find that they had stopped wearing the cap and cape she had so fallen in love with, but this is where her stories began. The funniest and saddest of times. From being given a pencil by her Grandad on graduation, saying "Use it when you need it Chick", to picking grown men off the floor after fainting at the sight of blood. Sarah-Anne's career was always exciting, working in A&E, acute surgery and growing into the role of Sister.

caps and capes. She graduated in 1995, only to find that they had stopped wearing the cap and cape she had so fallen in love with, but this is where her stories began. The funniest and saddest of times. From being given a pencil by her Grandad on graduation, saying "Use it when you need it Chick", to picking grown men off the floor after fainting at the sight of blood. Sarah-Anne's career was always exciting, working in A&E, acute surgery and growing into the role of Sister.

She then moved into a Nurse Practitioner role, diagnosing and prescribing, at the very beginning of what you see today in all GP surgeries. Then came her most wondrous challenge, supporting Jack, her eldest son through a painful period. He became her teacher, her master of how to use the weight of her words to support humans to see and hear themselves.

Birdonabike was born – Sarah-Anne's purpose, her reason to get up in the morning – to support women to believe in the health of their lives. Everyday 'Bird' feels blessed with magnificent women opening up their souls, sharing their vulnerability, their shame, and willing life to run through their bodies again. She is able to ignite their magic, to show them how to shine their light bright. She sees their worth where they choose to be blind; she knows what they choose to ignore; and she holds their faith where they have none. Sarah-Anne builds their beauty and strength from within until the path to unwavering faith is laid and they can wake up breathing into their power, standing strong throughout the day with an abundance of energy. Then they can create a ripple effect throughout their community and become their children's inspiration.

To find your unwavering faith head to Birdonabike.co.uk. Connect with Bird: the team love to hear from and support you. Birdonabike regularly hosts events and workshops throughout the year. Bird is giving away two free tickets to everyone who reviews this book.

Visit Birdonabike to see what's coming up... www.Birdonabike.co.uk.

If you would like to review this book, we will reward you for investing your time:

1. Write an amazing review of this book.
2. Post it on Amazon, your blog, Facebook page, everywhere possible.
3. Send a link or screenshot to Birdonabike.co.uk, with the heading 'Review'.
4. You will be sent two free tickets to a UK workshop. If you are not in the UK, check out the website for the international workshops being held and come along. It's a must that you come and say hello when at the event.

Set yourself apart.

Printed in Great Britain
by Amazon